DISCARD

DEMCO

The Lupus Handbook for Women

Up-to-date Information on
Understanding and Managing
the Disease Which Affects
1 in 500 Women

Robin Dibner, M.D., and Carol Colman

A Fireside Book
Published by Simon & Schuster
New York London Toronto Sydney Tokyo Singapore

FIRESIDE
Rockefeller Center
1230 Avenue of the Americas
New York, New York 10020

FIRESIDE and colophon are registered trademarks of
Simon & Schuster Inc.

Designed by Hyun Joo Kim

Manufactured in the United States of America

10   9   8   7   6

Library of Congress Cataloging-in-Publication Data

Dibner, Robin.
The lupus handbook for women : up-to-date information on
understanding and managing the disease which affects 1 in 500
women / Robin Dibner and Carol Colman.
   p.   cm.
"A Fireside book."
Includes bibliographical references.
1. Systemic lupus erythematosus—Popular works.
2. Women—Diseases. I. Colman, Carol. II. Title.
RC924.5.L85D53   1994
616.7'7—dc20   94-17984
                                                   CIP

ISBN: 0-671-79031-5

In memory of Ruth Rosenblum

Acknowledgments

I have had outstanding rheumatologists as teachers and mentors: William Clark, M.D.; Ellen Ginzler, M.D.; the late David Kaplan, M.D.; and Robert Lahita, M.D. They have always been generous with their knowledge.

I have been most fortunate that the SLE Foundation, the largest chapter of the Lupus Foundation of America, introduced me to Carol Colman, a wonderful writer whose knowledge and dedication have so impressed me.

I have had loving support from friends, family, my husband, Bruce, and our daughter, Sylvie.

My greatest teachers have been the many women (and a few men) with lupus I have known. They have taught me about courage and grace as they strive to lead life to the fullest.

I would also like to thank Lisa Sammaritano, M.D., and Laura Robbins, ACSW, both with the Hospital for Special Surgery, and Enid Engelhardt, CSW, of the SLE Foundation for their help with this project.

Contents

Introduction

I am a rheumatologist. Rheumatologists are clinicians and researchers who specialize in the care of patients with arthritis and other connective tissue diseases such as lupus. These diseases are characterized by destructive changes in the joints, muscles, tendons, and ligaments. There may also be changes in blood vessels throughout the body from damage caused by the immune system.

Since I was four years old, I knew that I wanted to be a physician. My interest in chronic disease developed in my early teens after I was diagnosed with Crohn's disease, a chronic inflammatory disease of the bowel. Although I am fine now, I was intermittently quite sick in high school and college and during my medical training. However, having to cope with the uncertainty of a chronic illness early in life has given me some insight into what my patients may be experiencing, and that is one of the reasons I chose a specialty that treats chronic illness.

I also became interested in treating people with lupus and other autoimmune diseases because they are often young patients, ones in whom effective treatment can have a real impact. I feel it is very important to help people with chronic illnesses live as fully as they are able, and that is one of the reasons why I wrote this book.

Many patients have explained to me their frustrations at not understanding their illness or treatment. Yet many say that they were too shy to ask a question, to "bother" their doctors or to express what might be misinterpreted as distrust of their doctor's advice or treatment. I hope that when you read this book, some of your questions will be answered. I also hope that you will appreciate how complex and individual each patient with lupus is.

Many questions remain unanswered, both for you and for the dedicated researchers in this field. We must work together to combat ignorance about lupus, increase public awareness, and support the much needed research that I am confident will answer many of our questions in the future.

The Lupus Handbook for Women is not designed to replace physician care, rather the goal is to educate patients so that they can work better with their physicians. Although there is no cure for lupus, good treatment and a cooperative effort between physician and patient can make a tremendous difference in the prognosis.

—ROBIN DIBNER, M.D.

CHAPTER 1

What Is Lupus?

At one time, lupus was considered a rare disease, but, thanks to better diagnostic techniques and greater awareness on the part of physicians, we now know that is it far more common than we ever thought. About five hundred thousand Americans have lupus, and more than 90 percent of these are women. About sixteen thousand new cases are diagnosed each year. (Asian, African-American, and Hispanic women appear to be at somewhat higher risk for lupus than Caucasian women.) Notably, lupus is more widespread than many better-known diseases, such as leukemia or multiple sclerosis. Lupus typically strikes women of childbearing age—usually between fifteen and forty—however, it can also occur in very young girls and postmenopausal women. In rare cases, infants of mothers with lupus or other connective tissue diseases may be born with neonatal lupus, a transient form of the disease that usually disappears within six months.

> I woke up one morning with a strange pain shooting from my neck down to my shoulders. I felt a lot more tired than usual. I went to see my doctor who decided

to test me for "the Three L's": Lyme disease, lupus, and leukemia. The tests were negative for all three, so he decided to treat me for Lyme and put me on very high doses of antibiotics. I went away on vacation and did a lot of sunbathing. I got a bright red rash all over my face, even in my scalp, and I was sore and puffy everywhere. When I came back, I went to another doctor, this time a rheumatologist, who took one look at me and said, "You don't have Lyme disease, you have lupus."

—Sarah, thirty-three

I was feeling ill with all kinds of funny symptoms. I'm normally very active, but I felt exhausted. It was a weird kind of exhaustion. No matter how much I slept, I still felt tired. I felt achy, I had floating arthritis. A joint would hurt one day, and then another joint would hurt the next day. Another strange thing—I couldn't close my jaw. It felt as if my dentist had put a filling in the wrong way. I went to an orthopedist and he said, "Well, you must have strained yourself lifting something." I went to another doctor, who tested me for Lyme, and I tested positive. My brother, who is a doctor, didn't believe that I had Lyme. He sent me to a rheumatologist, who ran all kinds of tests. She finally told me that I had lupus.

—Claire, fifty-one

All through high school I was sick. I had seizures, and my parents were told that I had some kind of seizure disorder. In my twenties, I began developing strange neurological symptoms. I thought I was having a nervous breakdown. I had difficulty focusing for very long periods at a time, and I had strange feelings in my head. I went to a doctor who suggested that I see a psychiatrist. I went to a psychiatrist, and after talking with me, he said that I was totally sane but terribly sick. He re-

ferred me to a rheumatologist, who told me that I was
having a lupus flare.

—Susan, thirty-seven

These three women experienced vastly different symptoms.
Yet, all three have been diagnosed with the same disease: systemic
lupus erythematosus (SLE), commonly called lupus, a chronic, inflammatory disease that can affect any part of the body. Like
many other women with lupus, these women were initially misdiagnosed and had to go from doctor to doctor before getting the
correct diagnosis, usually from a rheumatologist. Their experiences are echoed by hundreds of other patients. In fact, it is the
rare lupus patient who gets diagnosed quickly.

Although there is a growing awareness about lupus within the
medical community as well as among laypeople, a great deal of ignorance remains. Many cases go undetected or are misdiagnosed.
Part of the problem may stem from the lack of emphasis on diseases such as lupus in general medical education. Lupus is very
complicated, and because it is such a varied disease, it may be difficult to pigeonhole for medical students. In the past, rheumatology was covered only briefly in medical school, and lupus may
have been discussed in only one or two lectures (if at all) and usually only in connection with kidney disease. Although many medical schools now include more on rheumatology in their curricula,
the American College of Rheumatology (the professional organization of rheumatologists) has deemed it necessary to develop cur-
ricular materials to promote more in-depth coverage of
rheumatology in medical school.

To add to the general lack of awareness, lupus is not the kind of
disease that captures the constant attention of the media the way
that acquired immunodeficiency syndrome (AIDS) and to a lesser
extent breast cancer and Lyme disease have. Although it is not
known exactly how lupus is contracted, it is believed that it is not
contagious. Thus, public health officials do not feel that it is necessary to bombard the media with information on how to prevent
lupus as they do with AIDS or Lyme, because as far as we know,
lupus cannot be prevented. Second, unlike breast cancer, lupus
cannot be detected through a simple test such as a mammogram.

In fact, there is no single diagnostic test for lupus. And since women are not routinely screened for lupus, it is not a disease that is on the minds of most patients or even their physicians.

Lupus is also primarily a woman's disease. Historically, diseases that afflict women have been neglected by the medical establishment. In fact, to compensate for this neglect, the National Institutes of Health have recently mandated that women must be included in all research studies. Currently, in comparison to other "women's diseases," however, lupus has received more attention from researchers because of its link to the immune system, which is an area of science that has received much attention in recent years. Even so, there are few controlled clinical trials involving human subjects, and much more research is required in this and other areas pertaining to women's health.

Because most lupus patients are women, there is a risk that physicians may not take their complaints as seriously as they do those of male patients. Many women with lupus say that their complaints, at least initially, were dismissed by their physicians as unimportant. In some cases, vague symptoms such as fatigue or general achiness are quickly labeled psychosomatic, especially if the patient is female. The medical establishment has a long history of dismissing women's symptoms as "hysterical" or "neurotic," and there are many studies that document that this attitude may still prevail.

However, I believe that ignorance and sexism are not the primary reasons why women with lupus frequently have difficulty getting a correct diagnosis. In fact, the real culprit may be the quirky nature of the disease itself. There is no typical case of lupus. In some women, lupus may begin as a rash—often triggered by sun exposure—and quickly develop into serious kidney disease. In others, lupus may cause fatigue and arthritis. In others, lupus causes chest pain, hair loss, or cold hands and feet. In still others, seizures and Alzheimer's-type symptoms may be present. In many cases, patients may have difficulty articulating their symptoms because they cover such a broad range. When asked what's wrong, they often reply, "Everything hurts," or "I feel achy all over." They may be accurately describing how they feel, but this kind of vague response can confuse physicians or make them wonder whether the patient is overreacting. (Those of us who routinely treat lupus patients understand that our patients really do hurt all over.)

The diversity of lupus symptoms is mind-boggling, and as I mentioned earlier, to complicate matters even further, there is no one medical test that can positively confirm a diagnosis of lupus. Lupus can easily be mistaken for other diseases, such as Lyme (for which lupus patients often test false positive), chronic fatigue syndrome, and even depression. In fact, to clarify which patients should be considered to have lupus, the American College of Rheumatology developed a list of eleven criteria. A patient fulfilling four or more criteria usually has lupus. (These criteria are discussed in Chapter 2, see p. 27.)

THE COMMON LINK

Although every case of lupus is different, there is one common link: the immune system. Lupus is an auto(self)immune disease. This means that the strange and disparate symptoms characteristic of this disease are caused by a malfunction of the patient's own immune system. In a normal immune system, the body produces substances called *antibodies* to fight against germs or toxins (antigens) that could cause disease. These antibodies are usually careful to attack only the unwelcome invaders without harming healthy tissue. In lupus, however, the immune system becomes hyperactive: It begins producing excess quantities of antibodies that are directed against the body's own tissues—*autoantibodies*. Depending on the severity of the disease, these autoantibodies and cells that are part of the immune system attack different parts of the body. For example, some autoantibodies may be directed against the bone marrow, inhibiting production of red blood cells, which can cause severe anemia. Others can form substances called *immune complexes*, which can cause inflammation and damage many parts of the body. Connective tissue—materials between the bone and the muscles, including tendons, collagen, and cartilage—appears to be especially vulnerable to inflammation. Even major organ systems, including the heart, lungs, kidneys, eyes, and brain, can be damaged by these immune or inflammatory processes.

Although a hyperactive immune system seems to be the common link among lupus patients, that is where the similarity ends.

Some patients produce a large quantity of different antibodies, others produce very few antibodies. In fact, to add to the complexity, there is often no clear connection between the amount or type of antibodies that are produced and the severity of the symptoms.

THE DIFFERENT FORMS OF LUPUS

The term *lupus* refers to three different autoimmune diseases: discoid, SLE, and drug-induced lupus.

DISCOID LUPUS

Discoid lupus is a skin disease that is characterized by a rash that usually appears on the face, neck, and scalp and inside the ears. In most cases, discoid lupus does not cause other symptoms and does not affect any internal organs. However, if untreated, it can cause permanent scarring and baldness. About 10 percent of all cases of discoid lupus will develop into a mild form of SLE.

SYSTEMIC LUPUS ERYTHEMATOSUS

SLE, the most serious form of this disease, may involve the skin, joints, and tendons (connective tissue) as well as other body organs. Because of the involvement of connective tissue, SLE is often referred to as a *connective tissue disease*. However, lupus is also called a *collagen vascular disease* because inflammation of the blood vessels, vasculitis, is a common complication.

DRUG-INDUCED LUPUS

Certain drugs, notably hydralazine, which is used to treat hypertension, and procainamide, which is used to treat irregular heartbeat, can trigger lupus attacks in people who have no history of the disease. Usually, once the drug is discontinued, the symptoms gradually disappear. There is a genetic predisposition for drug-induced lupus, which is related to the way that medication is metabolized in the body.

THE PROGNOSIS IS GOOD

When the doctor said I had lupus, my mother cried. She had an aunt who had died very young from lupus many years ago. My doctor said that, for one thing, things had gotten a lot better and, for another, we shouldn't believe any horror stories that we heard about lupus. Just because something bad happened to someone else doesn't mean that my case is going to be like hers. As it turned out, my case has been pretty mild.

—Kelly, twenty-nine

Until recently, SLE—the most serious form of this disease—was considered fatal. A famous study conducted at Johns Hopkins University in the 1950s revealed that less than 50 percent of all lupus patients were alive after a mere four years following diagnosis. In recent years, that grim prognosis has dramatically changed for the better. Although lupus is a chronic disease and there is no cure, there are now a wide variety of highly effective treatments. In fact, depending on the study, it has been found that anywhere from 76 to 90 percent of all patients diagnosed with lupus will live ten years or more after diagnosis, and many will live normal life spans. With good medical care, most will have mild cases and live fairly normal lives. In most cases, even those who have severe recurrent attacks, or "flares," can be managed successfully. Unfortunately, women of lower socioeconomic groups have the worst prognosis, possibly related to their limited access to appropriate care.

THE CAUSES OF LUPUS

For centuries, the medical community has been baffled by this atypical and unpredictable disease. Unlike infectious diseases such as AIDS or Lyme, which are transmitted in specific ways, we don't know why or how people develop lupus or even why it is more common among women than men. We do believe that lupus is not contagious. We're not even sure if all the different symptoms that we label as lupus are actually caused by the same thing. Although we are far from having all the answers, we do have some intelligent theories about the possible causes of this disease.

Hippocrates may have been the first physician to describe lupus when he referred to a mysterious rash that appeared on the cheeks and nose in a distinctive pattern. The skin disease was named lupus in 1851 by a French physician who, believing that the bright red rash resembled the bite of a wolf, dubbed the disease *lupus* (Latin for wolf) *erythematosus* (Latin for red). In 1895, a renowned physician, Sir William Osler, recognized that some forms of lupus involved more than just a rash and actually affected internal organs, and he added the word *systemic* to the name.

THE IMMUNE SYSTEM

Very little was known about the possible causes of lupus until 1957, when researchers discovered the presence of autoantibodies in the blood of lupus patients. The discovery was provocative: Researchers now knew that a malfunction of the immune system was somehow involved in the disease process, but they still didn't understand the precise mechanism. Through the years, further study of immunity has shed some light on the workings of this complex and intricate system. Researchers now believe that the defect in the immune system that triggers the production of autoantibodies may be a result of a breakdown in communication between specific cells. Here is a much simplified explanation of their findings. Certain white blood cells called *lymphocytes* are key players in the production of antibodies. The B lymphocytes produce antibodies as the body needs them. Some T lymphocytes are called the *helper cells* because they promote immune responses and encourage the B lymphocytes to produce more antibody, and different T lymphocytes, known as *suppressor cells*, inhibit immune reponses and tell the B lymphocytes that it is time to cut back on production. Some researchers believe that for an unknown reason, in active lupus, the suppressor T cells fail to keep the brakes on the producer B cells, which throws the entire immune system out of balance and leads to the reckless production of autoantibodies. Interestingly enough, studies show that during active phases of the disease, lupus patients do not produce enough suppressor T cells. However, during the inactive phases, or times of remission, they have a normal amount of suppressor cells.

The immune system is extraordinarily complicated, and we still have much to learn about the mechanisms within the immune system that go awry causing lupus. At this point, we can only speculate as to why it happens. The current belief is that lupus may be caused by the complex interaction between several factors, including a genetic predisposition and specific environmental triggers.

GENETICS

There appears to be a genetic predisposition to develop lupus as well as other similar autoimmune diseases. However, the genetic link is somewhat complicated. About 10 percent of all cases of lupus are familial, that is, the patient has a close relative (parent or sibling) who also has lupus. Only 5 percent of children born to a parent with lupus will actually develop lupus. Research shows that people with particular genetic tissue types called *human leukocyte antigen* (HLA types) are more prone to develop lupus than those with other types. (Tissue types can be determined by a blood test.) HLA is genetically determined and related to immune function. There is also an increased incidence of lupus among identical twins (twins with the same genes), but only a slightly increased risk among fraternal twins, who are no more genetically connected than any other pair of siblings.

Interestingly enough, there is a somewhat higher rate of lupus among nonrelated members of the same household, such as stepsisters, than in the general population, which suggests that environmental triggers may also play a role. However, there is even a greater risk of nonrelated members of the same household developing autoantibodies without necessarily developing lupus.

This also suggests that some environmental factor—a virus, perhaps, or exposure to some chemical or medication—may trigger the production of autoantibodies. It seems likely though that only individuals who are genetically predisposed to lupus may actually develop the disease.

INFECTION

Many researchers strongly suspect that some as-of-yet unidentified infection may be responsible for the breakdown in communication between the T-helper cells and the B lymphocytes. We know that another disease that afflicts the immune system—AIDS—is caused by the devastating effect of a human immunodeficiency virus (HIV) that deactivates the immune system. It seems logical that a disease that has just the opposite effect on the immune system, which makes it hyperactive, may also be caused by a viral infection.

HORMONES

Many doctors believe that there is a connection between the female hormone estrogen and lupus, although we don't know exactly what it is. We do know that lupus tends to strike women at a much higher rate than men, usually after puberty when female hormone levels rise. We also know that high-estrogen birth control pills can trigger a flare in some women and that some women may experience flares during pregnancy, when all levels of female hormones, including estrogen, are higher than normal. Several studies have shown that neither men nor women with lupus metabolize or break down estrogen in the same way as people without lupus. Other studies have shown that estrogen may somehow activate the immune system, while androgens (male hormones) may somehow deactivate the immune system.

Finally, studies involving strains of mice prone to lupus demonstrate that female mice develop lupus earlier than male mice and have more severe cases. Related studies show that if the testes of male mice are removed, they will develop lupus earlier, whereas if the level of their male hormones is raised, the onset of lupus is delayed. As of yet, no one has conclusively found the link between estrogen and lupus, but it certainly bears further study.

THE SILICONE CONTROVERSY

Recently, there has been much publicity suggesting that breast implants made of silicone gel may trigger autoimmune diseases in women, including lupus, rheumatoid arthritis, and scleroderma, a connective tissue disease characterized by the thickening of the skin. Researchers have found that after silicone breast implantation, some women developed autoantibodies and/or symptoms of connective tissue disease. Moreover, it appears as if women who had ruptured implants or implants that leaked experienced symptoms sooner and more severely than those whose implants remained intact.

It is still unclear as to whether the silicone gel actually triggered these abnormalities or whether these women would have developed these problems anyway and the silicone merely accelerated the process. A third possibility is that these women would have developed autoimmune diseases whether or not they had implants. Until further studies can solve this mystery, many physicians believe that breast augmentation of any kind should be approached with extreme caution.

THE SYMPTOMS OF LUPUS

Although every woman with lupus may experience the illness in a different way, there are some common symptoms.

∾ FATIGUE. Of all the symptoms of lupus, fatigue is the most universal. Patients don't just complain about being tired, they talk about a form of deep exhaustion that interferes with their ability to function at anywhere near normal levels. I often hear things from patients like, "I used to be able to walk for miles, now I have to sit down after one block," and "I never used to take naps in the afternoon, now I can't get through the day if I don't." Many rheumatologists now believe that the fatigue and achiness in some lupus patients is compounded by another condition called *fibromyalgia*. This is a poorly understood syndrome characterized by fatigue, diffuse achiness, and certain characteristic tender points on physical examination. Although fibromyalgia syndrome is also seen in nonlupus patients, recent studies show that it may be present in nearly half of all lupus patients.

∾ PAIN. Patients often complain of almost flulike aches and pains all over their bodies. In some cases, patients describe a feeling similar to the muscle soreness that may occur after a vigorous workout. Some patients have arthritis, specific pain, and/or swelling in their joints, usually in the smaller joints in the hands and feet. Very often, they may wake up feeling stiff and uncomfortable. The pain may subside during the day and worsen at night.

∾ RASHES. A varity of rashes can be seen in lupus, but the most common is a red facial rash called *malar* or *butterfly rash*.

∾ SUN SENSITIVITY. A majority of women with lupus will have some symptoms (rash, fever, or achiness) after intense sun exposure.

∾ HAIR LOSS. During periods of active disease, patients may notice more hair on their pillow when they get up in the morning or more hair in the shower drain. Patches of hair loss may also be noted.

∾ FEVER. Some women with lupus run a low-grade fever of around 100 degrees all the time, and some develop a high fever that may come and go. The fever may increase at night.

∾ CHEST PAIN. A sharp pain caused by the inflammation of the lining of the heart or lungs is a common symptom of lupus.

❧ COLD HANDS AND FEET. About 20 percent of all women with lupus have Raynaud's syndrome, a sensitivity to cold in the fingers and often the toes. When exposed to cold, the fingertips can turn white and the nail beds can turn a bluish color. When rewarmed, the fingers become red. Raynaud's can be very uncomfortable, causing a deep, tingling feeling in the hands and feet. Emotional stress can also trigger episodes.

❧ DEPRESSION. Many lupus patients experience a severe, organic depression characterized by a sense of helplessness and hopelessness.

❧ EDEMA OR SWELLING. For some patients, the first sign of lupus may be swelling in the ankles and legs or around the eyes. Swelling can be a sign of kidney disease caused by the lupus.

❧ EASY BRUISING. Patients may notice that they bruise more easily, a sign of low platelet count (platelets are clotting cells that may be destroyed by autoantibodies).

❧ DRY EYES, DRY MOUTH. Many women with lupus have Sjogren's syndrome, in which autoantibodies attack the glands that produce saliva and other lubricants.

❧ PREMENSTRUAL FLARES. Many women report that whatever symptoms they have get worse right before their periods.

MANAGING LUPUS

Although lupus cannot be cured, it can be managed, most often quite successfully. The patients who fare the best—physically and emotionally—are the ones who, early on, become active partners with their physicians in managing their illness. Before this goal can be achieved, patients must come to terms with having lupus.

When someone is diagnosed with a chronic disease, the initial reaction is typically one of denial and anger. This is particularly true for many newly diagnosed women with lupus, who, as young adults, are planning on pursuing careers and starting families and do not want to be hampered by the physical constraints of chronic illness. There's a tendency to think, If I just ignore this, it will go away. However, in the case of lupus, denying symptoms such as fatigue, pain, and fever can be a terrible mistake. Prompt medical attention can often mean the difference between controlling the illness early on or developing a major flare. There are several steps that a patient must take in order to effectively manage her disease.

❧ EDUCATE YOURSELF. Knowledge is empowering. Learn about lupus. Contact the Lupus Foundation, the Arthritis Foundation, or any other resource group that can enhance your understanding of what's happening to your body (see Resources for addresses and phone numbers). An educated patient will be able to talk with her physician on a more sophisticated level and, more important, will be better prepared to be involved in the critical decisions about appropriate treatment.

❧ DEVELOP SELF-AWARENESS. Learn to know yourself. Become sensitive to your body. In particular, learn to recognize what's normal and what's not. It's your responsibility to report any significant change in symptoms to your physician as promptly as possible. (For more information, see Chapter 5.)

❧ AVOID SELF-BLAME. Patients need to learn that there are things that they can control, like maintaining a healthy lifestyle, watching for any unusual symptoms, and complying with their treatment regimens. However, even the most conscientious of patients can have a flare. I have seen too many women who have taken excellent care of themselves suddenly get ill and then blame themselves. They rack their brains, trying to figure out what they ate or what they did that could have triggered the flare. They are putting themselves through unnecessary grief. Some lupus patients suddenly flare for no apparent reason. No one is to blame, least of all the patient. You simply have to accept the fact that this disease is unpredictable and conserve your energy for getting better.

❧ DREAM YOUR DREAMS. You have a chronic disease that may require special attention, but your life is far from over. Although your disease is part of your life, it is not all of your life. Lupus not-withstanding, if you are truly motivated to do something, you should at least try to do it. There may be times when your illness interferes with your progress; dreams may have to be postponed or even modified. But I guarantee that you will bounce back faster and survive the challenges of chronic illness better if you keep your goals and dreams alive.

CHAPTER 2

Getting a Correct Diagnosis: Understanding the Tests and the Numbers

> I had joint pain, headaches, and fever on and off for three years, but my lab tests were normal. My doctor kept saying, "We know that something is going on here, but we can't say what it is." Finally, I developed a positive ANA [blood test] and some other abnormalities that led my doctor to believe that I had lupus. It may sound strange, but I was relieved to hear that there was actually something physically wrong with me, and it had a name. You begin to think that maybe you're imagining it, and you know that there are other people who think that your problem is all in your head.
>
> —Anne, twenty-nine, recently diagnosed with SLE

There is no one symptom or one medical test that conclusively points to a diagnosis of SLE. Therefore, a physician must carefully evaluate each patient to determine whether her particular combination of symptoms, laboratory results, and physical findings warrant a diagnosis of SLE.

A thorough and meticulous examination by a physician is a critical first step in establishing a diagnosis. Specific blood tests may also help to confirm the diagnosis. Although some cases may be very obvious—an experienced physician may be able to diagnose SLE at the initial visit—most cases are a lot trickier, even for the most skilled of practitioners. Other illnesses that have features similar to lupus must be considered. In fact, physicians have called lupus a "great imitator" because of the wide range of conditions it may mimic. Depending on the patient's symptoms, these may include other connective tissue diseases, such as rheumatoid arthritis, and infectious diseases, such as Lyme, syphilis, tuberculosis (TB), mononucleosis, and even AIDS. Doctors also have to rule out blood disorders, such as leukemia and lymphoma; neurologic disorders, such as multiple sclerosis; and psychiatric disorders, such as schizophrenia. In addition, lupus can look a lot like chronic fatigue syndrome and fibromyalgia, both of which are characterized by extreme fatigue and diffuse pain and both of which are poorly understood. (Nearly half of all lupus patients may have fibromyalgia at some point.) Much to a patient's frustration, it could take months or even years before the physician can rule out the other possibilities and say with any certainty, "You have lupus."

This chapter will explain how a physician may diagnose SLE, the various laboratory tests that may point to lupus, and perhaps, more important, the role the patient may play in helping her doctor evaluate her case.

THE ELEVEN CRITERIA FOR SLE

In all likelihood, to determine if you have lupus, your doctor has referred to the Criteria for SLE (officially known as the Revised Criteria for the Classification of Lupus, developed in 1982 by the American College of Rheumatology). It is a list of eleven abnormalities that are most specific for SLE. Some of the abnormalities on the list may also apply to patients with other autoimmune or connective tissue disorders as well as other unrelated diseases. As a rule of thumb, if a patient has had four or more of the eleven criteria (she doesn't need to have them all at once), she can be diagnosed as having SLE.

Before reading this list, rest assured that few patients ever develop all eleven abnormalities. Also, keep in mind, when it comes to SLE, there are few hard and fast rules. A skilled physician who is experienced in treating SLE patients may be able to make a diagnosis based on family history, the patient's symptoms, and physical examination even if she does not fulfill four of the eleven criteria. There are also some patients with four criteria who do not have lupus. Other diagnoses must still be considered and ruled out.

The following list outlines the eleven criteria and explains the role each plays in reaching a diagnosis of SLE.

∽ 1. MALAR RASH. About half of all SLE patients eventually develop the malar, or butterfly-shaped, rash over the cheeks and bridge of the nose. The folds of the nose are unaffected. The rash usually consists of red, raised bumps that may itch or be uncomfortable. However, on some patients, it will appear more like a red flush. The malar rash may be hot to the touch and may worsen during periods of active disease. For some patients, the rash may be milder in the morning and flare up later in the day.

Although the precise cause of the malar rash is unknown, it appears on the parts of the face that are most exposed to the sun, suggesting that the sun may trigger or at least aggravate the rash. In addition, biopsies of these rashes show that there are significant deposits of antibodies in the dermis, the deep layer of skin, as well as inflammation of blood vessels, which suggests an autoimmune response is also at play.

The malar rash may disappear either spontaneously or with treatment and does not cause any scarring.

∽ 2. DISCOID RASH. The discoid rash, which affects about 25 percent of all SLE patients, consists of discrete, round, scaly spots that often appear on the face but can also be on the arms, upper back, scalp, and ears. Discoid rash resembles psoriasis. However, unlike psoriasis, if you remove the scale of discoid rash, underneath it looks like a cluster of little blackheads. (The psoriasis lesion is red.) If untreated, the discoid rash can leave scars.

Discoid rash affects skin pigmentation: If you're fair skinned, the rash can leave a dark spot; if you're dark skinned, it can leave a white spot. If the rash appears on the scalp, it can result in permanent hair loss called *scarring alopecia.*

The discoid rash may also be aggravated by sun exposure and tends to worsen during spring and summer. Similar to malar rash, a biopsy of discoid rash reveals inflammatory cells in the affected areas.

Discoid lupus, in which the patient only has discoid rash and does not have any other organ involvement, is a separate disease and should not be confused with SLE discoid rash. However, about 10 percent of all patients with discoid lupus will eventually go on to develop SLE.

❧ 3. PHOTOSENSITIVITY. Most SLE patients are photosensitive, that is, they are sensitive to the sun and other forms of light. The exact relationship between photosensitivity and SLE is not fully understood. One theory is that the sun might damage the deoxyribonucleic acid (DNA) in the skin, which in turn makes the DNA appear to be abnormal to the immune system. Thus, the immune system makes autoantibodies to DNA, which may lead to inflammation and tissue damage. Typically, sun exposure will trigger a rash but could also result in fever, fatigue, joint pain, and other symptoms of SLE. In some cases, sun exposure could even cause the onset of kidney disease.

Both ultraviolet (UV) A and UVB rays are problematic for SLE patients. At one time, sunscreens only offered protection against UVB, the "burning rays," but now most also shield against UVA, the "tanning rays." Many lupus patients are also sensitive to light emitted from fluorescent bulbs (UVB) and halogen lamps (UVA).

❧ 4. ORAL ULCERS. As many as 40 percent of all SLE patients may have small erosions that resemble cold sores and are typically found on the hard palate of the mouth. Oral ulcers, which are caused by inflammation, are usually painless, and the patient is often totally unaware of them.

❧ 5. ARTHRITIS. Most SLE patients will suffer from a form of arthritis that does not damage bones but can cause swelling and inflammation of joints and ligaments, especially in the hands (particularly the knuckles), the wrists, and toes. Larger joints may also be involved. Arthritis symptoms may be transient or chronic and will often worsen during periods of active disease.

❧ 6. SEROSITIS. At least half of all SLE patients have serositis, the painful inflammation of the delicate linings covering the lungs, heart, or the abdominal cavity. Pleuritis occurs when the lining of the lungs becomes inflamed and can result in chest pain, especially when breathing in. Pericarditis is the inflammation of the tissue surrounding the heart and may also cause similar chest pain. Very often, this pain may become more acute when lying down and improve when sitting or leaning forward. Upon physical examination, a doctor may hear an abnormal sound called a *rub*, which suggests that there is inflammation and sometimes a buildup of fluid around the heart or lungs. These conditions may also be detected by a chest X ray; an electrocardiogram (EKG), a noninvasive test that measures the heart's electrical activity; or an echocardiogram, a noninvasive test in which sound waves are bounced off the heart to provide a picture of the structure of the heart.

Peritonitis, which occurs less frequently than pleuritis or pericarditis, is the inflammation of the lining of the abdominal cavity and can result in acute abdominal pain. It is often difficult to distinguish between the pain of peritonitis and appendicitis.

❧ 7. RENAL DISORDER. Most SLE patients have some form of kidney abnormality ranging from the leaking of protein into the urine (often a fairly mild condition) to the breakdown of the kidney's ability to remove toxins from the blood (a severe impairment). However, only about half will suffer permanent kidney damage. Usually painless and symptomless, kidney disorders are often detected after a urine analysis reveals an abnormally high level of protein or the presence of white or red blood cells, which are all signs of inflammation. Kidney involvement in lupus is often associated with high blood pressure (hypertension).

❧ 8. NEUROLOGIC ABNORMALITIES. About 50 percent of SLE patients develop problems of the central nervous system (CNS) at some time. About 25 percent of all patients have neurologic problems at the time of diagnosis. Involvement of the CNS in SLE can cause a wide range of disorders, from acute seizures and pyschosis to chronic forms of confusion and memory loss. Seizures are epileptic episodes in which the patient may black out and the body goes into convulsions. Psychosis, a condition in which thinking and behavior become abnormal, may manifest itself in the form of a severe, organic depression or as schizophrenic-type symptoms, such as hallucinations and bizarre behavior.

∞ 9. HEMATOLOGIC ABNORMALITIES. There are four hematologic abnormalities, or disorders of blood cells, that are often found in SLE patients but may also be a sign of another problem. They are caused by autoantibodies that attack particular kinds of blood cells. Following are the major forms of blood disorders in lupus that are included in the criteria.

(a) *Hemolytic anemia.* The patient makes antibodies against her own red blood cells, which causes their removal by scavenger cells in the spleen or liver. If untreated, hemolytic anemia may be very serious.

(b) *Thrombocytopenia.* This condition is characterized by a low number of platelets, or clotting cells (less than 100,000 platelets per cubic millimeter), which is caused by autoantibodies that destroy these cells in the spleen. A severe drop in platelets can result in bleeding.

(c) *Leukopenia.* The white blood cell count is low (below 4,000 cells per cubic millimeter). This is usually not a serious condition but may indicate the lupus is active.

(d) *Lymphocytopenia.* The lymphocyte count is low, which is not considered to be serious and rarely by itself impedes the body's ability to fight infection.

Any one of the these four blood abnormalities (or combination of them) counts as 1 point toward the eleven diagnostic criteria.

∞ 10. IMMUNOLOGIC ABNORMALITIES. There are four antibodies that are found in the blood that when combined with other symptoms may suggest a diagnosis of SLE.

(a) *Anti-DNA antibodies.* Many SLE patients produce antibodies against their own DNA or genetic material.

(b) *The lupus erythematosus cell preparation (LE prep).* The LE cell is found in the blood of 90 percent of patients with active SLE. However, it may also be found in patients with other autoimmune disorders including rheumatoid arthritis, scleroderma, and Sjogren's syndrome. The first laboratory test designed to detect SLE, the LE cell test is not as specific as some of the more recent tests and is no longer widely used.

(c) *Antibodies to Sm (Smith)*. These autoantibodies, named after the patient in which they were first identified, are directed against a protein found in the cell nucleus. Between 30 and 40 percent of all SLE patients have antibodies to Sm. The anti-Sm antibody test is highly specific for SLE, meaning that it is extremely rare that it would be found in people with other disorders. Therefore, if you test positive for anti-Sm antibodies, you are likely to be diagnosed with SLE.

(d) *A false-positive serologic test for syphilis*. About 20 percent of SLE patients will test positive for syphilis, although SLE is totally unrelated to this or any other venereal disease. Certain SLE patients produce antibodies that can be similar to those produced by a patient trying to fight off syphilis, hence, the positive test. Syphilis also causes inflammation of blood vessels and many other symptoms that are similar to SLE. Great care must be taken to distinguish between the two if the syphilis test is positive.

Any one of the above immunologic abnormalities counts as 1 point toward the eleven criteria.

～ 11. ANTINUCLEAR ANTIBODIES (ANA). About 95 percent of all lupus patients test positive for ANA, that is, autoantibodies to cell nuclei. However, a positive ANA may also be found in patients with other autoimmune disorders as well as people taking certain medications and even in some completely symptomless, healthy people. Therefore, a positive ANA test by itself does not make a valid diagnosis of lupus. However, it can point to SLE if it is accompanied by characteristic SLE symptoms, physical exam findings, or other test results, such as a positive anti-DNA or anti-Sm test.

ANA test reports provide two pieces of information: a titer and a pattern. The titer is a number that tells how many times a patient's blood must be diluted to obtain a sample that is free of ANA. A titer of 1:80 is usually, but not always, considered positive. Lower titers are not usually significant. The higher the titer, the more antibody that is present in the blood. The ANA titer may vary during the course of the disease and does not necessarily reflect the severity of the condition.

The pattern refers to the way the autoantibodies arrange themselves. The ANA pattern may help differentiate SLE from other conditions that may cause a positive ANA result. The smooth, homogenous pattern is often found in patients who are taking certain medications, who have a connective tissue disease, or who are healthy despite the positive ANA. The speckled pattern is most often found in SLE and other connective tissue diseases. The peripheral pattern or rim is usually found only in SLE.

IN THE DOCTOR'S OFFICE

Only five of the eleven criteria for determining a diagnosis of SLE rely on numbers obtained from laboratory tests. The rest can only be determined by information obtained through the interaction between a patient and her physician. The following outlines the important role that both must play to help reach a diagnosis.

THE FAMILY MEDICAL HISTORY

Perhaps the most important part of the doctor's examination is the exchange of information between patient and doctor. At the initial meeting, the physician will usually ask for a medical history of your family to determine if there could be a genetic predisposition to a particular problem. Be prepared to give him or her the appropriate information. For example, if you're suffering from arthritic-type pain or extreme fatigue, check to see if a close blood relative (a parent, sibling, grandparent, aunt, or first cousin) has ever experienced similar symptoms or had ever been diagnosed with a related disorder. Even if you're not prepared to do this for your first meeting, once your doctor suggests that you may have a connective tissue disease, you may be able to check with your relatives to see if anyone else may have had a similar problem. Keep in mind that seemingly unrelated illnesses, such as kidney disease, high blood pressure, arthritis, or blood clots, could be valuable clues in helping your physician make an accurate diagnosis.

PERSONAL MEDICAL HISTORY

Be prepared to give your physician a brief but concise list of your current symptoms. In addition, you should make him or her aware of past medical problems including a list of previous surgical procedures, blood transfusions, allergies, serious illnesses, fevers, skin rashes, or unexplained hair loss. Also tell your doctor if your symptoms get worse after any particular activity or during any part of the day. (Very often, with SLE, patients feel worse later in the day or when they are fatigued. Patients with arthritis may feel stiff or sore in the morning upon waking.)

Be sure to tell your doctor if you have taken any medication or have had any infection in the past. For example, you may not think that it is relevant to mention that you were recently put on medication for a bladder infection, yet some of the drugs used to treat that problem have been implicated in triggering flares in lupus patients. Since SLE can be triggered by several drugs and possibly by certain infections, it is extremely important to tell your doctor this information.

Few people would consider talking about their vacations as part of their medical history, yet it can be invaluable information when dealing with SLE. I've had several patients whose symptoms began after they had returned from Caribbean vacations, where they spent their days soaking up the sun. Because photosensitivity is a sign of SLE, let your doctor know if you've been exposed to the sun recently, even if just for a day.

Give your doctor an accurate account of your gynecological history. Let him or her know if your menstrual status has recently changed or if you are currently or have ever taken birth control pills or estrogen replacement therapy—hormones are believed to play a role in SLE. Also, be sure to tell your physician if you've had a history of miscarriage; certain antibodies found in some SLE patients can cause spontaneous abortion or stillbirth.

THE PHYSICAL EXAMINATION

In addition to a good routine physical examination, including a check of blood pressure and weight as well as a review of all vital organs, your physician will also take extra care in looking for the telltale signs of SLE and other related diseases.

Hair Loss: Your physician will examine the scalp for signs of hair loss or scarring from a discoid rash.

Eye Examination: Your physician may do an examination of your eyes with a fundoscope to look at the back of the eye for signs of cytoid bodies, evidence of blood vessel inflammation that is related to CNS disease.

Ulcerations: Your physician will check for any oral or nasal ulcers, painless erosions on the hard palate or in the nose that the patient may not even know about.

Lymph Nodes: Swelling in the lymph nodes can be a sign of inflammation. Therefore, your physician will palpate areas around your neck, above the collarbones, in the armpits, above the elbows, and in the groin.

Thyroid Gland: The thyroid gland is located at the front of the neck. Your physician will check for enlargement of this gland, which may be a sign of an underactive thyroid sometimes seen in lupus.

Skin: Your physician will look closely at your skin for active rashes or evidence of scarring from a discoid rash, particularly in the ears. Very often, I find that a patient may have had a discoid rash and might not have even known it or may have mistaken it for something else. All that remains is the telltale scar, which can provide important information for the doctor.

Chest Examination: Your physician will listen to your chest with a stethoscope for evidence of pleuritis, inflammation of the lining around the lung, or pericarditis, inflammation of the lining around the heart. He or she will also check for fluid, another sign of inflammation.

Organ Enlargement: Your physician will palpate your liver and spleen for evidence of swelling, a sign of inflammation.

Edema: Your physician will check for edema or fluid in the lower legs. This could be a sign of kidney disease, which can occur in SLE.

Joints: Your physician will palpate the joints for signs of tenderness and swelling. In patients with lupus arthritis, the joints will usually be tender upon touch.

Abnormalities in Fingers or Toes: Discoloring (blueness) or other abnormalities of the fingers or toes can be a sign of SLE-related problems such as Raynaud's syndrome. In some cases, your physician may do a nail-fold capillary examination in which he or she puts a drop of oil at the edge of the cuticle and looks with a magnifier to reveal certain abnormalities of the blood vessels.

Neurologic Exam: Your physician will do a careful neurologic exam to make sure that your sensation, reflexes, and muscle strength are normal. This is very important, because it may alert the physician to any problems involving the CNS.

LABORATORY TESTS

In many cases, your physician will be able to reach a diagnosis on the basis of family history, personal medical history, and the physical examination. In some cases, however, he or she may still not be able to pinpoint the particular disease or disorder. In either case, your physician will probably call for other laboratory tests in addition to the ones that are normally performed to either verify a suspected diagnosis or to obtain more information.

When SLE is suspected, the physician will usually order the following laboratory tests.

   ✎ COMPLETE BLOOD COUNT (CBC). Your blood cells can tell a great deal about your overall health. First, about half of all SLE patients have a low white blood cell count. Most will have a low red blood cell count. Low red blood cells is a sign of many chronic illnesses and, in some cases, is called the anemia of chronic disease. A small number of SLE patients will develop hemolytic anemia in which they are producing antibodies against their own red blood cells, which also results in a low red blood cell count. Another 15 percent of SLE patients have thrombocytopenia, a lower than normal level of platelets. Any or all of these abnormalities in blood cells could be a sign of SLE.

   ✎ BLOOD CHEMISTRY SCREEN. A blood chemistry screen tests for many different levels of chemicals and enzymes in the blood. However, when SLE is suspected, the physician is most interested in the tests that measure for kidney function. The creatinine level measures how well the kidneys are purifying blood; the BUN (blood urea nitrogen) also measures the level of renal function. In addition, the physician will check the serum albumin level, which shows how much of this protein is in the body. If the protein level is significantly below normal, it is likely that damaged kidneys are leaking albumin into the urine.

   ✎ URINANALYSIS. The physician will look for protein in the

urine or for red or white blood cells scattered or in clumps called *casts*, all of which are signs of inflammation of the kidney.

⮂ SEDIMENTATION RATE (ESR). This test is a very nonspecific test that is used as a general screen to determine whether there is an inflammatory disease. People who have active inflammation will usually have an elevated ESR. However, it can also be elevated in most infections and tumors as well as other connective tissue diseases.

⮂ ANA. This is a screening test for autoantibodies to cell nuclei in the blood. However, patients with many other related problems or those taking certain medications may also have a positive ANA. In addition, people who have absolutely no symptoms may test positive for ANA, in which case, the test results should be ignored until or unless any symptoms arise. A negative ANA test suggests that the patient may not have SLE. Less than 5 percent of all lupus patients do not test positive for ANA; however, virtually all of them will show some other abnormal antibodies.

⮂ RHEUMATOID FACTOR (RF). If a patient has arthritic symptoms, the doctor may test for RF. About 75 percent of patients with rheumatoid arthritis test positive for RF; however, only 20 percent of patients with lupus test positive. Patients with lupus who are RF positive tend to have milder cases of lupus.

⮂ SEROLOGIC TEST FOR SYPHILIS. A false positive for this test is one of the immunologic criteria for establishing a diagnosis of lupus. Roughly 20 percent of SLE patients will test false positive for syphilis.

⮂ LYME TITER. The symptoms of Lyme are similar to those of SLE. Therefore, it is important to rule out the possibility of Lyme disease before diagnosing a patient with SLE if she has been in an area where Lyme is frequently seen. The screening test is called an ELISA (enzyme-linked immunosorbent assay). Unfortunately, SLE patients can have a false-positive result for Lyme disease on the ELISA and, therefore, may require a more specific follow-up blood test called a *Western blot*.

⮂ HIV TEST. Although they are very different illnesses, many of the manifestations of AIDS can be confused with those of SLE. Mouth ulcers, facial rashes, hair loss, swollen lymph nodes, low white blood cell counts, fever, and protein in the urine can all be signs of either illness. Patients who have been sexually active or who have other AIDS risk factors should be tested for HIV. Because a false-positive ELISA test for HIV can be seen in SLE and other conditions, the labs routinely follow up any positive result with the more specific Western blot blood test. Very often, SLE patients will be put on immunosuppressive drugs, which is exactly opposite of the treatment for HIV and could accelerate the undiagnosed or misdiagnosed AIDS patient's demise.

After this first round of tests, your doctor may have enough information to make a diagnosis. However, in some cases, more highly specific tests may be necessary to rule out other connective tissue diseases. Even if your doctor is convinced that you have SLE, he or she will probably order additional tests to obtain a "serologic fingerprint" at the time of diagnosis. From this additional blood data, your doctor can often predict complications that may arise down the road and can alert you to watch out for particular changes in your condition.

■ TEST FOR ANTI-DS (DOUBLE-STRANDED OR NATIVE) DNA ANTIBODIES. Many SLE patients produce antibodies to their own DNA or genetic material. Antibody to DNA is one of the immunologic criteria for establishing SLE. The test for anti-ds DNA antibodies is positive in roughly 70 percent of all SLE patients. It is rare for antibodies to ds DNA to be present in diseases other than lupus. They are more often found in SLE patients with active disease or kidney disease.

■ TEST FOR ANTI-SM (SMITH) ANTIBODIES. The antibody to this particular protein found in the cell nucleus is one of the immunologic diagnostic criteria. This test is very specific for lupus.

■ ANTIBODIES TO RIBONUCLEAR PROTEIN. These antibodies are common to SLE and other related disorders. Often, women with nonspecific lupuslike symptoms who do not fulfill the criteria for SLE will have high levels of antibodies to ribonuclear protein. These women may be diagnosed as having mixed connective tissue disease, overlap syndrome, or undifferentiated connective tissue disease and may or may not later develop SLE.

■ ANTIBODIES TO RO AND LA (ANTI-SSA/RO, ANTI-SSB/LA). These particular autoantibodies can be found in 30 to 40 percent of all SLE patients as well as in people with other autoimmune diseases. Because these autoantibodies can cause complications during pregnancy, it is important for women of childbearing age to know if they test positive. They are most often positive in patients who have dry eyes and dry mouth (Sjogren's syndrome).

  ANTIPHOSPHOLIPID ANTIBODIES. Antiphospholipid antibodies are directed against certain phospholipids, a family of fat molecules that are widely distributed in the body. Although many SLE patients have these antibodies, there are also many people with antiphospholipid antibodies who do not have SLE. Some may have clotting problems and others appear to be perfectly healthy.

There are several types of antiphospholipid antibodies, but there are two that are most associated with SLE: the lupus anticoagulant and anticardiolipin antibodies.

There are different blood tests used to detect the lupus anticoagulant and anticardiolipin antibodies. A blood-clotting test known as the *activated partial thromboplastin time* is often used to screen for the lupus anticoagulant.

An ELISA test is used to measure anticardiolipin antibodies, of which there are several different classes (IgG, IgM, IgA). High titers of IgG anticardiolipin seem to be more closely associated with excessive blood clotting.

Women with either the lupus anticoagulant, anticardiolipin antibodies, or both—the so-called antiphospholipid antibody syndrome—are at risk of developing clotting problems that could include heart attack, stroke, and deep venous thrombosis (leg clots). In addition, they may be more prone to miscarry as are non-SLE women with antiphospholipid antibodies.

  SERUM COMPLEMENT LEVELS. Complement is a family of proteins in the blood involved in fighting infection and inflammation. People with active SLE tend to have lower than normal complement levels. The combination of a low complement and a high level of antibodies to DNA may indicate a patient at greater risk of developing kidney disease. In some patients, complement levels are followed over time and may predict flares.

THE NONSPECIFIC DIAGNOSIS

There are times when even after a thorough examination and a battery of laboratory tests your doctor is not able to make a concrete diagnosis. You may be experiencing one or two symptoms—fever and a rash, or Raynaud's syndrome and fatigue—that could suggest any number of connective tissue diseases, including SLE. Your test results may reveal some evidence of inflammation and autoimmune activity. However, based on your symptoms and the laboratory findings, it is virtually impossible to identify the specific problem. In these cases, your doctor may say, "You have some kind of autoimmune disease, and we have to wait and see what happens to determine which disease it becomes."

Many patients may be frustrated by a vague diagnosis; they would prefer to know exactly what is wrong. However, their physicians really do have their best interest at heart. It's a mistake to prematurely label a patient, especially when that label may be wrong. For one thing, it's very difficult to convince an insurance company that a diagnosis was a mistake; that inaccurate label could follow you around for a lifetime. More important, physicians who diagnose too quickly could close their minds to the possibility that their patient does indeed have some other kind of connective tissue disorder or disease that may require a completely different type of treatment. In these cases, it is far better to err on the side of caution.

WHEN TO GET A SECOND OPINION

Getting to a diagnosis of SLE is a lot different than getting to a diagnosis for many other ailments. For example, in the case of cancer, the proof is in the biopsy. In most cases, a physician can render a definitive diagnosis of cancer based solely on laboratory tests. Not so with SLE. A diagnosis of SLE is often a judgment call on the part of the physician. Every patient deserves an in-depth explanation from her physician as to why he or she has made the diagnosis. In some cases, a patient may feel completely comfortable with her doctor's explanation and may not look any further. Other patients, however, may want to seek a second opinion. It is within the patient's right to do so. In fact, in many cases, if the primary physician is an internist or family practitioner, he or she may automatically refer a newly diagnosed SLE patient to a rheumatologist for confirmation of the diagnosis.

Getting a second opinion is one thing; the practice of "doctor hopping" is another. When a patient is diagnosed with a chronic and unpredictable disease such as SLE, there is a temptation to search for the doctor who can offer a panacea or quick fix. Many patients change doctors frequently in their attempt to find a cure. This is unwise and can have dangerous ramifications. It is important for an SLE patient to forge a relationship with one physician who will be responsible for her primary care. It is extremely important to be monitored by a doctor who knows you well enough to discern any subtle changes in your condition. When it comes to SLE, early intervention can often make the difference between a minor problem and a major emergency.

At times, depending on your symptoms, your primary care physician may call in other specialists. For example, he or she may consult a nephrologist if you develop kidney disease or a neurologist if you develop neurologic problems. It is critical for these specialists to work in tandem with your primary care physician.

FINDING A PRIMARY CARE PHYSICIAN

When you have a chronic disease such as lupus, choosing the right physician can be a decision of extreme importance. Ideally, you will develop a long-term relationship with one physician who will manage your case through the years. If you're already working with a doctor you like and trust, there's no reason to change. However, many women do not have a primary care physician; very often, they rely on their gynecologists to manage their health care. If you don't have a primary care physician, you need to find one. This can be a challenge. You need a doctor who is not only competent, but one you feel comfortable enough to call when you have a problem. You also need to find a doctor who is experienced with lupus and who keeps up-to-date on the latest research findings and treatments.

Here are some factors you need to consider in searching for the right doctor for you.

❧ WHERE DO YOU FIND ONE? There are several places where you can get referrals to competent physicians. Both the Arthritis Foundation and the Lupus Foundation will provide the names of physicians in your area who are skilled in treating lupus. If you attend a support group at the Lupus Foundation or the Arthritis Foundation, you can also get referrals from patients themselves. In addition, you can call your local hospital or medical research center for names of physicians who are specialists in rheumatology or who have experience with lupus patients. Your county medical society will also provide a list of local physicians with a specialty in rheumatology.

❧ CHECK OUT CREDENTIALS. Once you have a list of names, do some further checking. Find out how long the physician has been in practice and the type of specialty training she may have had. Does she have certification by the American Board of Internal Medicine and/or the American Board of Rheumatology? Although nothing can guarantee quality, and there are some fine physicians without these credentials, it is helpful to know if a physician has met the high standards set by these certifying professional organizations. Check the reference section of your local library for the *Official ABMS Directory of Board Certified Medical Specialists*, published by Marquis Who's Who. The county medical society may also provide this information, or you can call the doctor's office and ask the nurse or secretary.

Also be sure to find out how much experience the physician has had with lupus: Ask directly, "How many lupus patients has the doctor treated?" If the doctor doesn't have any other lupus patients in her caseload, she may not be that experienced in treating this disease. If the doctor does research in addition to seeing patients, find out how much of her time is devoted to patient care. Does she see patients only on certain days? What if you need to see her on another day? If your doctor's time is tied up in a laboratory, she may not have enough time for you.

❧ WHO COVERS FOR THE DOCTOR? If the doctor is unavailable, who covers for his patients? Does this physician (or physicians) have experience in lupus?

❧ HOSPITAL AFFILIATION. Be sure to find out with which hospital the physician is affiliated. You don't want to be forced to go to a hospital that may be second rate because that is where your doctor has admitting privileges.

❧ HOW THE OFFICE IS RUN. Before even making an appointment, check whether the style of the office is suitable to your lifestyle. What are the office hours? If you work outside the home or have children in school, you may need to make appointments at particular times. Find out if the doctor will make lunch-hour appointments or has hours on weekends or evenings. Even if a doctor has the best credentials in the world, it won't do you any good if you can't get in to see her.

❧ THE LENGTH OF APPOINTMENTS. Ask the secretary how much time the physician allocates for each appointment. For a disease as complicated as lupus, the physician should allow at least an hour for the initial visit. Follow-up appointments will take on average about fifteen to thirty minutes. (In some cases, if you have a lot of problems and need more time, you should alert the office ahead of time.) If the nurse or receptionist says that the physician allows only five to ten minutes per appointment, it's an indication that he may be very rushed.

❧ TELEPHONE POLICY. Ask the nurse or receptionist how the doctor handles questions in between visits. Does she have a special time set aside each day to answer questions? Will a nurse talk with you and then speak with the doctor on your behalf? Will the doctor only speak with you if it's a true emergency? These answers will give you some idea of how accessible the doctor is to her patients.

❧ FINANCES. If money is an issue, find out ahead of time the office policy on billing. Many doctors expect that the patient will pay the full bill at each appointment and that it is the patient's responsibility to collect from the insurance company. However, some physicians may accept payment from certain insurance plans or may be members of group insurance plans. (The passage of a national health insurance plan could dramatically change fees and billing procedures.)

From this preliminary investigation, you should be able to narrow down your list to a few names. Then, in order to make your final decision, you need to make an appointment to see the physician(s) for a consultation. At the initial interview, there are some additional factors to consider.

❧ GENERAL IMPRESSION OF OFFICE. Is the doctor's office pleasant and clean? Does it appear to be well run? Is there a comfortable area for the patients to wait? Are patients expected to routinely wait for more than a half hour even when the doctor does not have an emergency? If the wait between appointments is excessive, it could be a sign that the doctor is overbooking. Is the staff pleasant? Going to the doctor can be stressful enough without having to put up with unnecessary irritants.

❧ MEETING THE PHYSICIAN. Choosing a physician is very subjective. One person may prefer a doctor who is businesslike and professional, another may want a doctor who is very personable who will remember the names of her children and her pets. Whichever style you choose, keep in mind that you need a physician who is not off-putting nor one who is so busy rushing off to the next appointment that you feel that he's not even listening.

❧ STYLE OF CARE. You need to make sure that your physician will be willing to work with you in a true partnership to the degree you are comfortable. Your physician should speak to you as an intelligent, informed adult; answer your questions; and consider your suggestions. From the initial interview and the manner in which the physician speaks to you, you may be able to discern how the physician views her patients. If you have any doubts, ask directly, "How do you feel about patients participating in managing their own care?" The best response is, "I prefer to work with an involved, informed patient because I believe that it yields a better result."

❧ OTHER ISSUES. If there is anything else that you passionately care about, make sure that you and the prospective doctor see eye to eye. For example, some patients are adamant that they want their parent or spouse to be present during the examination. Some physicians may be equally adamant that they don't want anyone else present. If you have any strong feelings about these or other related issues, check them out with the doctor ahead of time.

CHAPTER 3

What Can Go Wrong

Many women with SLE have only mild symptoms, and although they may experience an occasional flare, most develop few serious medical problems. However, SLE can increase the odds of developing particular complications that can be very serious, especially if they are not treated promptly. The following chapter lists some of the most common complications and how they are diagnosed and treated. It is especially important for SLE patients to be familiar with the potential hazards of this disease; detecting a problem early is your best defense against developing major organ damage.

KIDNEY DISEASE

The purpose of the kidneys is to purify the blood of the body's waste products and to help maintain the normal fluid and chemical balance in the blood. The kidneys are among the most vulnerable organs in SLE. About one-third of all SLE patients will develop *lupus nephritis* (also known as *lupus glomerulonephritis*), a serious kidney disease that can lead to kidney failure. Many more SLE patients will have some form of mild kidney problem.

Kidney disease is particularly insidious because there are often no symptoms: It is possible for a patient to be close to kidney failure and not have an inkling that she is seriously ill. The signs of kidney disease, fatigue or swelling, can easily be mistaken for other illnesses or the usual symptoms of SLE. Therefore, it is critical for SLE patients to have their kidney function monitored periodically by their physicians with blood and urine tests.

SLE patients with a low complement level and a high anti-DNA seem to be especially prone to developing major kidney disease and need to be watched closely by their physicians.

High blood pressure may be one of the first and only signs of developing kidney failure. (A normal premenopausal woman has a blood pressure of between 110/65 and 120/80. Anything higher than 120/80 is considered above normal.) Uncontrolled hypertension can be devastating to the kidneys, rapidly accelerating the rate of failure. It's very important that your physician routinely check your blood pressure. If your physician prescribes any antihypertensive medication, take it according to instructions; not doing so could cost you your kidneys.

❧ SYMPTOMS

There are several subtle signs that could indicate the development of kidney disease. If you experience any of them, notify your doctor immediately.

Swelling. Swelling or edema around the eyes upon rising in the morning or around the ankles or shins could suggest a buildup of fluid, which could be an early sign of kidney failure.

Fatigue. If you've been feeling well and suddenly begin to feel extremely tired or if you're decidedly more fatigued than usual, check with your doctor. This could be a sign of kidney disease.

Nosebleeds. When the kidneys are failing, platelets don't work well and can result in bleeding, especially from the nose.

Foaming of urine. This can indicate that protein is leaking into the urine as a result of kidney damage.

Increased urination at night. An increase in the need to urinate at night and a decrease in urination during the day may be a sign of kidney failure. Blood flow is better to the failing kidney at night while lying down, increasing urine production.

Confusion. Patients experiencing kidney failure may become forgetful and confused.

Loss of appetite for meat. When the kidneys begin to fail, breakdown products of protein become toxic to the body. Nephrologists have noticed that patients often eliminate meat and other high-protein foods from their diets, almost as if they knew that their bodies could not tolerate these foods. Some believe, in these situations, a low-protein diet may delay kidney failure.

Nausea and vomiting. These symptoms could signify kidney disease as well as many other problems.

Chest pains. Severe kidney disease could cause pericarditis.

෨ DIAGNOSTIC TESTS

Blood tests. Blood levels of BUN and serum creatinine can determine how well the kidneys are purifying the blood of toxins. Other irregularities in blood chemistry may also signal a kidney problem and may themselves pose a danger, such as elevated potassium levels, which can cause cardiac rhythm irregularities.

Severe anemia could be a sign of kidney failure—the hormone that stimulates red blood cell production is located in the kidney. Once the kidney fails, it does not produce enough of this hormone.

Urine tests. Urine is tested for excess protein (proteinuria) or for signs of blood—either red blood cells (hematuria), white blood cells, or casts—which point to inflammation of the kidneys.

Imaging studies. Ultrasound (sonogram) can rule out any obstruction or structural abnormalities and can determine the size of the kidneys, which can indicate if the problem is acute or chronic.

Twenty-four-hour urine test. This test provides a more accurate assessment of kidney function than the one-time urinalysis by measuring the creatinine clearance and protein content in the urine over a twenty-four-hour period. The patient is asked to collect all urine over twenty-four hours. The test begins after the first urine of the day (which is discarded). Every drop of urine thereafter is collected in a container. The first morning urine of the following day is collected, which completes the test.

Kidney biopsy. Patients with strong evidence of kidney disease may need to undergo a kidney biopsy in which a small section of the kidney is removed, usually by a needle inserted through the back, and studied under the microscope to determine the type and severity of the disease. This procedure is done in a hospital.

෨ TREATMENT

Diet. Patients with kidney disease may be put on a low-salt, low-potassium, and/or low-protein diet.

Corticosteroids. Drugs such as prednisone, prednisolone, or methyl prednisolone are used to suppress the immune response that causes the kidney damage. Patients may be put on high doses of steroids, sometimes intravenously. Pulse steroid therapy—a high intravenous dose for three days and then oral steroids, gradually tapered down—has been shown to be effective in reversing acute deterioration of kidney function.

Immunosuppressive drugs. The chemotherapy drugs azathioprine (Imuran) and cyclophosphamide (Cytoxan) may be used to control severe organ damage.

Dialysis. If the kidney involvement does not respond to treatment and progresses to complete kidney failure, also called *renal failure*, the patient may require dialysis. In hemodialysis, a patient in renal failure is put on a machine that performs the job of the kidney: The blood is removed from the body, passed through filters where it is purified, and then returned to the body. This procedure takes about four hours and is usually performed three times a week, usually at a dialysis center. Peritoneal dialysis is a procedure that also effectively performs the job of the kidney. The advantage of peritoneal dialysis is that it can be done by the patient at home. In this procedure, fluid is placed in the peritoneum (the abdominal cavity) through a surgically implanted catheter. Impurities are then drained out through the catheter.

In some cases, SLE patients do not remain in permanent kidney failure. For some unknown reason, a number go into remission after hemodialysis. In fact, the other symptoms of SLE, including rashes, fatigue, and joint pain, seem to improve after the kidneys fail, especially in those treated with hemodialysis.

Kidney transplant. In cases of permanent kidney failure, kidney transplantation may be an option. Stable SLE patients are considered excellent candidates for this procedure and have fared very well afterward.

CARDIOPULMONARY COMPLICATIONS

SLE can lead to a variety of heart and lung problems that require specific treatments. About one-third of all SLE patients will develop some kind of a heart or lung complication.

PERICARDITIS

Pericarditis, fairly common to SLE patients, is the inflammation of the sac that surrounds the heart. In most cases, it is a relatively mild problem than can be easily treated.

SYMPTOMS

Chest pain. Generally, patients with pericarditis experience chest pain that may feel worse when they are lying down and better when they sit or lean forward. The pain usually starts in the middle of the chest and radiates to the back.

Shortness of breath. In severe cases, patients may have difficulty catching their breath.

Swelling. Edema or swelling in the legs could result in advanced cases.

DIAGNOSTIC TESTS

Abnormal sound. During an examination with a stethoscope, the physician may hear a rub.

EKG. An EKG, a painless test that measures the electrical activity of the heart, may detect an abnormality.

Echocardiogram. By bouncing sound waves off the heart, this noninvasive, painless test can produce a picture of the structure of the heart. It will show any fluid around the heart that may result from inflammation.

TREATMENT

The most common therapy involves using high doses of nonsteroidal anti-inflammatory drugs (NSAIDs) or corticosteroids over a short period of time.

MYOCARDITIS

This serious condition, caused by inflammation of the heart muscle, occurs in about 5 to 10 percent of all SLE patients.

SYMPTOMS

Chest pain. Pain or discomfort occurs across the chest that could be mistaken for a heart attack.

Shortness of breath. Similar to pericarditis, a woman with myocarditis may have difficulty catching her breath. The inflamed heart muscle is failing to contract adequately, which can result in heart failure and fluid buildup in the lungs.

Fever. A patient may run a fever as a result of the inflammation.

❦ DIAGNOSTIC TESTS

EKG. Myocarditis could resemble a heart attack or cardiac injury on an EKG.

Imaging. Nuclear cardiac scanning may reveal the inflammation in the heart muscle.

Echocardiogram. An echocardiogram will show the diffuse malfunctioning of the heart muscle.

❦ TREATMENT

Myocarditis is treated with high doses of corticosteroids or immunosuppressive drugs.

CORONARY ARTERY DISEASE

Coronary artery disease (CAD) is the result of a devastating process called *atherosclerosis*, in which the arteries bringing blood to the heart become clogged with plaque, a waxy, yellowish substance that impedes the flow of blood to the heart. As women with SLE live longer due to better treatments, we are beginning to see a higher incidence of CAD in later life. Although all postmenopausal women have a significantly higher rate of CAD than women who are still menstruating, the rate among SLE patients appears to be much higher than normal.

There are several reasons why women with SLE may be more prone to developing CAD. First, many SLE patients, especially those on steroids or with kidney disease, develop very high blood cholesterol levels, a major risk factor for CAD. Second, because the kidney helps regulate blood pressure, many women with kidney disease may develop high blood pressure, which significantly increases their risk of having a heart attack or stroke. (If you are hypertensive, it is critical that you and your physician work together to get your blood pressure down to normal levels either through diet, exercise, antihypertensive medication, or a combination of all three.) Third, many SLE patients may have suffered from vasculitis, or inflammation of blood vessels—in this case, the coronary arteries—which may have caused damage to those vessels in the past, thus predisposing them to the formation of plaque.

Finally, women with antiphospholipid antibodies (about one-third of all SLE patients have them) may be prone to clotting problems that could result in a heart attack if a blood clot is formed in the coronary artery or lodges there from some other point in the heart.

When it comes to CAD, prevention goes a long way in keeping the disease at bay. A healthy lifestyle—not smoking, getting enough exercise, a low-fat diet, and maintaining normal weight—is your best defense against developing atherosclerosis or having a heart attack.

❧ SYMPTOMS

Many women with CAD will experience no symptoms at all before having a heart attack. In fact, in women, in about one-third of all cases there were no warning signs or the warning signs were ignored. However, others may have some telltale symptoms that should not be ignored.

Angina. A heaviness or squeezing tightness in the chest that may radiate to the back, up to the neck, or down the arm.

Shortness of breath. A sensation of having difficulty breathing, or finding that you're huffing and puffing at the slightest exertion.

Feeling faint. A feeling of lightheadedness, or that you're going to pass out.

❧ DIAGNOSTIC TESTS

There are many tests used to diagnosis CAD. The most common are the following.

EKG. An electrocardiogram may be used to detect signs of injury to the heart muscle. However, it may not always detect CAD.

Echocardiogram. This sonogram of the heart may reveal signs of past injury to the heart, but cannot show whether the coronary arteries are diseased or narrowed.

Thallium stress test. The normal exercise stress test is often not accurate for women. Therefore, many women are asked to take the thallium stress test. In this procedure, a radioactive substance is used to trace the flow of blood through the heart after the patient has exercised to a predetermined heart rate. This test can diagnose CAD with 90 percent accuracy in women.

Cardiac catheterization. This test, which is done under local anesthesia in a hospital, involves injecting a dye into the heart through a catheter to trace the blood flow through the coronary arteries throughout the heart.

❧ TREATMENT

There are many different treatment options for coronary artery disease—from medication to surgery—and any woman who has been diagnosed with a problem should consult with a cardiologist to determine her treatment options. However, there are some treatments that are commonly prescribed.

Cutting cholesterol. Patients with abnormally high cholesterol levels (for women, a fasting level of over 230 milligrams per deciliter) may need to reduce their cholesterol through dietary change or medication. Gemfibrozil has been used to lower cholesterol in women with SLE with good results. Many other drugs, including niacin (a form of vitamin B), may be useful under your doctor's supervision. Lovastatin, a widely used antilipid drug, should only be used with great caution in women with SLE; there have been several cases of drug-induced lupus caused by this medication. The antimalarial drug hydroxychloroquine, which is widely prescribed for SLE, can also produce a modest reduction in cholesterol but is not used to treat high cholesterol.

Antihypertensive medication. I can't stress this enough: It is critical for SLE patients to keep their blood pressure within normal limits. High blood pressure is called the silent killer because there are few if any symptoms. Some women may not see the need to take medication for a problem they cannot see or feel, especially if they are taking other drugs for SLE. However, high blood pressure is a very real disease and must be treated.

Vessel repair. If the coronary arteries are irreparably damaged to the extent that the heart is not getting enough blood, the physician may suggest balloon angioplasty or bypass surgery. In balloon angioplasty, a guiding catheter with a balloon on the end is inserted through an arm or leg to the place where the artery is narrowed by obstruction. The balloon is then inflated, flattening the plaque against the artery wall, thus opening up the artery. In coronary bypass surgery, a vein or artery from another part of the body is grafted from the aorta to a point below the obstruction on the artery, thus providing an alternate route for the blood to flow.

VALVULAR HEART DISEASE

There are four heart valves within the heart that open and snap shut to ensure that the blood flows in the right direction and doesn't back up. For years, it has been known the heart valves in lupus patients can become abnormally thick or develop wartlike growths called *Libman-Sacks lesions*. Until recently, these valve problems were poorly understood in women with SLE. We now believe that this condition is related to the antiphospholipid antibody syndrome, which may cause blood clots to form on the heart valves. Usually, these growths do not disturb the normal heart function. However, at times tiny emboli or pieces of the abnormal heart valves can break off and lodge in other parts of the body. Sometimes leaky valves may also result, causing a heart murmur.

❧ SYMPTOMS

Usually no symptoms. Shortness of breath may indicate a buildup of fluid in the lungs if the heart is unable to pump adequately due to leaky valves.

Palpitations. The patient may experience heart palpitations or an irregular heartbeat.

Persistent fever. A fever could indicate an infection on the abnormal heart valve, called *bacterial endocarditis*.

Stroke. If bits of the abnormal heart valve break off and enter the circulation of the brain, a stroke could result.

❧ DIAGNOSTIC TESTS

Physical exam. The physician may hear an abnormal sound or murmur.

Echocardiogram. This sonogram of the heart can trace the flow of blood through the nooks and crannies of the heart to detect any valvular abnormalities.

❧ TREATMENT

Antibiotic prophylaxis. If a valve lesion is diagnosed, the physician will recommend antibiotics before dental cleanings or major invasive procedures to prevent any bacteria released into the blood from infecting the valves.

Blood thinners. Aspirin or other blood thinners may be prescribed to reduce the risk of emboli from abnormal valves.

Valvular replacement. In rare and severe cases, cardiac surgery for valvular replacement may be necessary.

PULMONARY DISEASE

SLE can affect the lungs in any number of ways. The most common complication is pleuritis, the inflammation of the lining of the lung.

SLE patients on steroids or immunosuppressive drugs may be prone to develop lung infections such as bacterial pneumonia or fungal infections of the lung. If a patient had ever been exposed to TB, it could be reactivated if her immune system is depressed due to immunosuppressive medication.

In rare cases, a patient may develop lupus pneumonitis, an acute inflammation of the lung similar to severe pneumonia but actually caused by the SLE.

Patients with clotting disorders may develop a pulmonary embolus, that is, they throw a clot that lodges in the blood vessels of the lung. The first sign of the problem may be shortness of breath, chest pain, or coughing up blood.

Because there could be so many different causes, any lung problem needs to be carefully evaluated by a physician.

∞ SYMPTOMS

Chest pain. Pain of any kind could be a sign of a problem, but pain upon deep breathing is a characteristic symptom of pleuritis.

Difficulty breathing. Patients with lung ailments often have difficulty catching their breath and may have shortness of breath upon even mild exertion.

Coughing blood. Coughing up blood could be a sign of lung disease. Any bleeding should be reported to your doctor.

Cough with thick, discolored sputum. This symptom, especially if associated with fever or chest pain, suggests pneumonia. (Although a fever is usually present in cases of pneumonia, patients on immunosuppressive therapy who are most susceptible to infection may not have fever when infected.)

∞ DIAGNOSTIC TESTS

Physical exam. Using a stethoscope, the physician may hear a rub, which signifies inflammation, or other abnormal breath sounds due to infection.

Imaging. A chest X ray will show any fluid buildup around the lung, a sign of inflammation, pneumonia, and other physical manifestations of lung disease.

Lung scan. A radioactive substance is used to trace the blood flow through the lungs. The flow will be abnormal if there is a clot (pulmonary embolus).

Blood tests. In severe cases, the patient may undergo an arterial blood gas test, in which blood is obtained from an artery and is measured for oxygen, carbon dioxide, and the acid–base balance (pH) of the blood.

Sputum analysis. If an infection is present, the sputum will be analyzed in the laboratory to determine the cause of the infection.

Lung biopsy. If all else fails to diagnose the problem, lung tissue is obtained to review under the microscope.

♔ TREATMENT

Antibiotics. If an infection is diagnosed, antibiotics are prescribed.

NSAIDs or steroids. In cases of pleuritis, NSAIDs or steroids are given to reduce inflammation.

Blood thinners (heparin or coumadin). In pulmonary embolus these are given to prevent further clotting.

Immunosuppressive drugs. In cases of lupus pneumonitis, immunosuppressive drugs and/or steroids may be prescribed.

NEUROPSYCHIATRIC DISORDERS

Neuropsychiatric symptoms are caused by a wide range of medical or psychiatric disorders that may indicate SLE involvement of the nervous system, a highly complex group of specialized cells that transmit information throughout the body. The nervous system is divided into two parts: The central nervous system (CNS) encompasses the brain and the spinal cord and controls much of our behavior; the peripheral nervous system includes the nerves that extend to the edges of the body (arms, hands, legs, and feet).

Neurologic problems are one of the first manifestations of SLE in some patients. However, at one time or another, about half of all SLE patients will suffer from one or more of these disorders. Following are some of the more common forms of neuropsychiatric disease.

CENTRAL NERVOUS SYSTEM DISEASE

CNS disease is a very broad umbrella for a diverse group of problems ranging from epileptic-type seizures, memory loss, headaches, muscle weakness, confusion, clinical depression, and even psychosis. (Because depression is so common in SLE and a particular problem of women in general, it will be covered separately, see p. 58.)

CNS disease in SLE is still poorly understood, and it is often difficult to get a precise diagnosis. For one thing, although scientists suspect that the disease must somehow attack the portions of the CNS that control behavior, the exact mechanism is still unknown. For another, not every change in behavior is directly related to SLE. For example, symptoms such as forgetfulness, confusion, and dementia could be a result of extreme anxiety, an emotion not uncommon to women battling a chronic illness. Or these symptoms could be brought on by corticosteroids, which are widely prescribed for SLE. They could even be caused by an infection, especially if the patient is on steroids or other immunosuppressive medication.

To add to the confusion, recently many doctors have begun to suspect that in patients with antiphospholipid antibodies symptoms of CNS disease may actually be a result of small blood clots that cause tiny strokes in the brain.

Diagnosing CNS involvement can be a challenge to the most experienced of physicians—there is no definitive test for diagnosing CNS disease in SLE. Getting to the correct diagnosis can be as complicated as diagnosing SLE itself. If a patient develops neuropsychiatric symptoms, her physician must carefully evaluate her condition before prescribing treatment.

✤ SYMPTOMS

The symptoms for CNS disease are as varied as the disease itself. Patients should notify their physicians if they experience any of the following.

Headache. Severe or chronic headaches could be attributed to CNS disease from lupus, infection, or high blood pressure.

Epileptic-type seizures. Any episodes of convulsions, seizures, or abnormal involuntary movements could signify CNS disease.

Bizarre behavior. Delusions, loss of reality, hallucinations, or any signs of erratic behavior or abrupt behavior changes need to be reported to your physician.

Forgetfulness or confusion. Missing appointments, frequently stopping midsentence because you can't remember what you want to say, or forgetting something as simple as where you live could all be signs of a CNS problem.

Signs of stroke. Severe dizziness; dimming or loss of vision; persistent weakness or numbness in the face, arm, leg, or down one side of the body; loss of speech or confusion, and severe headaches could be a sign of a problem such as a stroke. If you have any of these symptoms, it is critical that you call your doctor immediately.

☙ DIAGNOSTIC TESTS

Imaging tests. The CAT scan (computerized axial tomographic scan) and magnetic resonance imaging (MRI) are noninvasive imaging tests that allow physicians to actually see how the brain looks. The MRI in particular is helpful because in addition to showing any area of bleeding, interrupted blood flow (infarct), tumor, or atrophy, it can show more subtle abnormalities of brain tissue that may have been caused by SLE.

Electroencephalogram (EEG). This painless, noninvasive brain wave test shows areas of abnormal electrical activity in the brain of patients with seizures or other neurologic involvement.

Psychometric testing. If a patient feels that she is becoming forgetful or is "losing it" in other ways, her physician may have her evaluated by a clinical psychologist who performs a battery of tests to measure cognitive function.

Spinal tap (lumbar puncture). In this procedure, a needle is inserted in the lower back to remove fluid from around the spinal cord, which is evaluated for signs of infection or inflammation.

☙ TREATMENT

Steroids and immunosuppressive drugs. If the physician has excluded steroids and infections as the cause of the symptoms, he or she may prescribe steroids or increase the dose if the patient is already taking this medication to suppress any SLE activity that may be causing the problem. In most cases, within a week or two, the patient will show improvement. Spontaneous improvement may also be seen in some cases. In severe cases of CNS disease, the physician may prescribe an immunosuppressive drug such as azathioprine (Imuran) or cyclophosphamide (Cytoxan).

Anticonvulsant drugs. Drugs such as phenytoin (Dilantin) and phenobarbital can help control seizures. (Although Dilantin may cause drug-induced lupus, it has been very widely and successfully used in treating lupus patients for CNS disorders.)

Antipsychotic drugs. Drugs such as haloperidol (Haldol) and thioridazine (Mellaril) are very helpful in treating psychiatric symptoms of lupus. Antidepressant drugs are also used.

Blood thinners. If the patient has a clotting problem that has caused a stroke or even multiple small strokes, her physician will prescribe a blood thinner such as aspirin, heparin, or coumadin.

Antibiotics. If the problem is traced to an infection (meningitis), antibiotics or antifungal treatment may be prescribed. Although meningitis is very serious, once the infection is under control, the patient usually returns to normal.

CLINICAL DEPRESSION

As many as one in five healthy women experience clinical depression at some point in their lives, and the figure is probably even higher for women with a chronic illness such as SLE. Clinical depression is not to be confused with feeling down or a little low for a few days or even a few weeks; rather it is a severe, often debilitating illness characterized by feelings of hopelessness and helplessness. People who have a true clinical depression are often unable to function normally and may be quite overwhelmed by their daily responsibilities.

Similar to other neuropsychiatric disorders, diagnosing the cause of depression can be extremely difficult. The depression could be physical in origin, somehow related to SLE's effect on the brain (the exact mechanism is still unknown) or other organs such as the thyroid. However, depression could also be an emotional response to the strain of having to cope with a difficult illness such as SLE, or it could even be caused by steroids. In some cases, depression could be a result of a combination of factors.

Fortunately, depression can be cured: Very often, patients improve within a few months with or without treatment. However, proper treatment may speed up the recovery process and even help prevent the depression from recurring. Although depression can be very disturbing, it is frequently overlooked by both patients and physicians. All too often, patients are reluctant to ask for help or are ashamed to admit that they have a psychological problem. Physicians who are focused on physical ailments may completely miss the subtle signs of psychiatric illness. Both physicians and patients may mistakenly believe that it's perfectly understandable to be depressed if you have a chronic illness. However, true depression is far from normal and should never be dismissed or ignored. It's very important for doctors of SLE patients to take a few moments during each visit to check up on their patient's mental state. It is also of critical importance for patients to share their thoughts and feelings with their physicians.

⮠ SYMPTOMS

Depressed mood. People who are clinically depressed are sad most of the time and often cry or feel like crying. They tend to feel like everything is hopeless and that life is not worth living. They may even become suicidal. They often lose interest in things that once excited them and may find that they are unable to concentrate.

Sleep disturbances. A change in normal sleep patterns, such as insomnia, excessive fatigue, or early morning wakening, could be a sign of depression. Because SLE patients often feel tired, a dramatic change in the level of fatigue could signify a problem.

Change in appetite. Excessive eating or undereating could be a sign of depression.

Physical ailments. Chronic pain, indigestion, headaches, and palpitations could be signs of depression. Because some of these symptoms are also typical of SLE symptoms, it's important for a physician or patient to try to sort out the SLE symptoms from possible depressive illness.

⮠ DIAGNOSTIC TESTS

Psychiatric evaluation. A physician, preferably one who is familiar with the patient, will carefully evaluate the patient for signs of changes in lifestyle or behavior that could point to depression. Evaluation by a psychiatrist is usually recommended, especially in severe cases, to help in diagnosis and guide treatment.

Blood tests. Thyroid function tests are essential to rule out the possibility that an underactive thyroid is contributing to or causing the problem. This problem is frequently seen in lupus patients and is easily treatable.

⮠ TREATMENT

Psychotherapy. In very mild cases, supportive psychotherapy may be adequate treatment without drugs. I believe the patient must be closely monitored by a mental health professional, that is, a psychiatrist or, in milder cases, a social worker or psychologist under a psychiatrist's (M.D.) guidance. The Lupus Foundation and the Arthritis Foundation have referral resources for psychotherapists experienced with SLE.

Antidepressants. This is an extremely effective family of drugs (brand names Norpramine, Prozac, Zoloft, Elavil, etc.) that boost the levels of chemicals in the brain called *neurotransmitters.* Patients usually begin to show significant improvement within two to three weeks.

Steroids. In severe cases, especially if the patient has a slowing of movement or thought, steroids may be tried.

SJOGREN'S SYNDROME

Sjogren's syndrome, also called *sicca* (dry) *syndrome,* is a chronic autoimmune, inflammatory disease in which the body's glands fail to produce enough protective lubricant, resulting in dry mouth (xerostomia), dry eye (keratoconjunctivitis sicca), and often vaginal dryness. (If Sjogren's is part of another illness, it is designated a syndrome; if it occurs by itself, it is called a disease.) Many patients with connective tissue diseases, such as SLE and rheumatoid arthritis, develop Sjogren's. As well as causing some discomfort, Sjogren's syndrome can lead to other more serious complications. For example, vaginal dryness can increase the risk of contracting a fungal or other type of infection. Dry eye can result in injury to the cornea, which can impair vision, as well as an increased risk of eye infection. Dry mouth can cause gum disease, tooth decay, cold sores, and other throat problems.

Certain medications, such as some antidepressants and antihypertensives, can exacerbate these problems. A doctor may consider changing medications if a patient develops any of these symptoms.

❦ SYMPTOMS

Dry eyes. The eyes may sting or burn, feel dry and gritty, and have thick mucus, especially in the morning.

Vaginal dryness. There may be vaginal burning or itchiness and great discomfort during sexual intercourse.

Dry mouth. The mouth and tongue may have a tacky, sticky, or dry feeling. It may be difficult to do simple things like lick a stamp. The patient may have swollen glands under her jaw or cheeks.

❧ DIAGNOSTIC TESTS

In most cases, patients can detect the symptoms of Sjogren's syndrome on their own and will alert their physicians.

Schirmer filter paper test. The physician may wish to confirm the diagnosis of dry eyes by performing this test to measure tear production.

Blood diagnostic tests. Lupus patients with Sjogren's are more likely to have two particular autoantibodies: anti-SSA/Ro and anti-SSB/La.

Biopsy. In the case of dry mouth, sometimes a minor biopsy of the lip (performed by an oral surgeon) is necessary to confirm the diagnosis.

❧ TREATMENT

Eye drops and ointments. Artificial or liquid tear preparations, steroid drops or steroid based ointments may be used to replenish the tear supply and reduce inflammation. Slow-dissolving moisture inserts that release liquid over time (Lacrisert) may be placed in the eye once a day. Lubricating ointments may be used at bedtime. Because they can cause blurry vision, they should not be used during the day.

Surgery for dry eyes. In a simple procedure, the ophthalmologist can surgically close off the tear duct that drains tears out of the eye, which can prevent whatever tears you do make from being drained off.

Mouth spray. If frequent sips of water don't work, the patient can use synthetic saliva sprays, which are sold over the counter. If that doesn't help, the physician may prescribe pilocarpine, an oral medication that helps to increase saliva production.

Vaginal lubricant. Over-the-counter vaginal lubricants, such as Replens, can offer great relief. Treatment of vaginal yeast infections, which Sjogren's patients are also prone to, will also reduce symptoms.

Medication. Corticosteroids or immunosuppressive drugs may be given orally to reduce inflammation in severe cases.

EYE DISORDERS

In SLE, the eyes can be affected in any number of ways. A common eye ailment, episcleritis, is the result of the inflammation of the outer layers of the sclera, the white of the eye. Scleritis, a more serious problem, is caused by a deeper inflammation in the eye and is relatively rare. Another possible problem is iritis, an inflammation of one of the interior chambers of the eye, which could result in blurred vision, light sensitivity, and a sore, red eye. Uncommonly, inflammatory cells can damage the blood vessels that supply the retina, resulting in small retinal hemorrhages that can prevent blood from flowing to the retinal tissue. In other cases, a blockage of blood flow to the optic nerve could result in blindness in that eye.

Sjogren's syndrome (see p. 60) can cause dryness and inflammation, which can lead to infection and damage of the cornea. Some of the medications used to control SLE can also cause eye problems. High doses of steroids taken long term may promote glaucoma and the formation of cataracts. The antimalarial drug chloroquine taken at high doses over a long term may cause vision loss. The newer antimalarial, hydroxychloroquine (Plaquenil), is believed to be safer; however, there is still a risk of eye damage, albeit a small one.

❦ SYMPTOMS

Red eye. Red, sore, swollen eyes or sensitivity of the eyes to light could indicate an eye infection or some other problem.

Vision disturbances. Any change in vision or blurring of vision could be a sign of an eye problem.

Discharge. Mucus or discharge from the eye could be a sign of infection.

❦ DIAGNOSTIC TESTS

Lupus patients should be evaluated by an ophthalmologist yearly to check for eye involvement with a dilated examination of the fundus (to check the retina) and slit lamp examination for inflammation in the eye (iritis). The ophthalmologist should also check for glaucoma and cataracts as well as color and peripheral vision for patients on antimalarials.

❦ TREATMENT

Antibiotics. If the problem is due to infection, antibiotics may be prescribed either orally or in the form of eye drops.

Steroids. Problems due to inflammation, such as iritis or episcleritis, may be treated with steroid eye drops.

(For treatment of dry eye, see p. 93.)

ORTHOPEDIC COMPLICATIONS

Avascular necrosis is a relatively common complication associated with SLE, and affects the hip joint. Although the exact cause of the condition is unknown, it appears as if the small blood vessel that feeds the hip joint becomes occluded (blocked), resulting in an inadequate blood supply into the hip. The cartilage of the hip joint gets inadequate nourishment and dies; eventually the bone under the cartilage also dies and collapses. Over time, the loss of the cartilage can lead to a very severe degenerative arthritis. This condition is associated with steroid use and antiphospholipid antibodies. In some cases, early intervention may be helpful, so symptoms should be reported to the doctor immediately.

✿ SYMPTOMS

Early on, the patient may feel sharp pain in the groin or buttocks or have few symptoms. Later, she will have painful limited motion of the hips.

✿ DIAGNOSTIC TESTS

An MRI, a noninvasive procedure that uses powerful magnets to image the inside of the body, can detect avascular necrosis long before it shows up on a conventional X ray.

✿ TREATMENT

Medication. NSAIDs are used to treat pain and inflammation.

Surgery. In early cases, orthopedic surgeons sometimes attempt to decrease the pressure in the head of the hip bone with varying success. In severe cases, patients may need total hip replacement surgery.

CHAPTER 4

Treatments for Lupus

CONVENTIONAL DRUGS AND THERAPIES

The prognosis for SLE patients has dramatically improved over the past few decades in part because of an array of effective drug therapies. These medications not only help to control SLE symptoms but in many cases may also prevent or substantially delay the severe and often disabling organ damage that can curtail the quality and duration of life for some women with SLE. The vast majority of SLE patients do very well on most of these medications and experience few problems. However, there are potential risks to any medical treatment. This chapter outlines both the benefits and risks of each medication.

Please do not be discouraged by the possible side effects listed for each drug—the risks of not taking your medication for fear of side effects usually far outweigh any potential risk incurred by taking it. However, there are many different medications to choose from, and if you experience any untoward side effects from one, your physician has the option of prescribing another.

NONSTEROIDAL ANTI-INFLAMMATORY DRUGS

By far, NSAIDs are the most commonly prescribed drugs for SLE. These are usually the drugs of choice for patients with mild SLE with little or no organ involvement. Patients with more severe problems may take these drugs in addition to others.

There are many NSAIDs, the most common being aspirin (acetylsalicylic acid). Other NSAIDs include ibuprofen (Motrin, Advil, and other brands) and naproxen (Naprosyn), among many others.

Although they fall into several different chemical classes, all the NSAIDs are similar and work like aspirin. NSAIDs work by inhibiting the production of prostaglandins, substances that are mediators during the inflammatory process. Unlike drugs such as acetaminophen (Tylenol), NSAIDs are not merely analgesics (pain killers). What makes these drugs unique is that they actually reduce the signs and symptoms of inflammation. These drugs are quite effective in relieving joint and muscle pain, reducing fever, and sometimes even help in relieving fatigue.

Not every NSAID is going to have the same effect on every person. If you don't respond well to one drug, you may respond better to another. In addition, patients may do very well on one particular NSAID for a few months or even a year, and then, for some unknown reason, the drug becomes ineffective. Quite often, simply switching to a different NSAID can once again produce a beneficial effect.

The usual dosage varies with each drug. Some are designed to be taken once a day, and others as often as four times a day. Some people may prefer long-acting medication that can be taken only once a day. Although long-acting medications are very effective, others may prefer the psychological benefit of taking their medicine several times daily as a direct response to their pain.

ఆఅ SIDE EFFECTS

Gastrointestinal problems. Although prostaglandins can cause inflammation in other parts of the body, they protect the stomach lining against irritation. As a result, NSAIDs can cause symptoms and problems ranging from mild stomach upset (gastritis) to ulcers to the more serious gastrointestinal bleeding. Taking these drugs along with food can help prevent stomach distress. If you suffer from an upset stomach, nausea, vomiting, heartburn, or blood in the stool or vomitus, report it at once to your physician. It could be a sign that you are developing gastritis or an ulcer from NSAID use. In some cases, your physician may prescribe a drug called misoprostol (Cytotec), which helps replace the lost prostaglandins in the stomach and has been shown to be effective in decreasing the risk of NSAID-induced gastrointestinal damage or irritation.

If you are at risk of developing ulcers, that is, you have had gastrointestinal problems in the past, are elderly, or smoke, your doctor may consider putting you on misoprostol as a preventive measure. Most physicians are hesitant to prescribe misoprostol to women of childbearing age as it can cause miscarriage, so other medications may be given, including antacids (Maalox) or other drugs known as H_2-receptor blockers (Tagamet, Zantac, and other brands), which block acid production in the stomach. Another medication, Carafate, puts a protective lining in the stomach. The overall effectiveness of these treatments in preventing ulcers from NSAID use has been somewhat disappointing, but many patients find that their symptoms do improve.

Because of the risk of gastrointestinal bleeding, if you are taking an NSAID, your stool should be chemically tested for occult (hidden) blood periodically.

Bleeding. Aspirin as well as many other NSAIDs suppress the function of platelets or clotting cells in the blood, which can make you more prone to bruising or bleeding anywhere in the body. (Nonacetylated salicylates [Disalcid, Trilisate] do not have this effect on platelets.) If you're on an NSAID that can cause a bleeding problem, discontinue the drug a few days before having any dental work or major surgery. In the case of aspirin, you will need to discontinue taking it at least two weeks ahead of time. (Of course, check with your physician before stopping this or any other prescribed medication.) Anyone who is on a blood thinner or who has a bleeding disorder such as hemophilia will need to be very carefully monitored on an NSAID or should be put on another medication.

Chronic low-grade blood loss from the stomach (gastritis, ulcer), if undiagnosed, could result in iron deficiency anemia. This

could be distinguished from other anemias of SLE (hemolytic anemia and anemia of chronic disease) by testing for iron levels in the
body. Testing the stool for blood will help distinguish this from
iron deficiency caused by excessive menstruation.

Decreased blood flow to the kidneys. Prostaglandins help keep
the arteries to the kidneys dilated and the blood flowing. Therefore, if you take a drug that blocks the action of prostaglandins,
you may inadvertently reduce the blood flow to the kidneys. For
most people, this is not a problem; however, if you have kidney
disease, you should use these drugs with caution. If you're on an
NSAID, your renal function should be routinely monitored.

Liver toxicity. Some lupus patients may develop hepatitis due to
a toxic response in the liver to aspirin or NSAIDs. Involvement of
the liver by lupus itself is not common. Therefore, it is imperative
to routinely monitor liver function in patients on these drugs.

Allergies. Some patients may be allergic to aspirin; typically,
these patients have asthma and nasal polyps. These patients are
probably at risk of developing an allergy to any drug in this class
and should be put on different medication or very carefully monitored if they are taking any NSAID.

Aseptic meningitis. NSAIDs may precipitate aseptic meningitis,
a form of noninfectious meningitis that looks very much like the
infectious variety—the patient develops headaches, neck stiffness,
eye sensitivity to light, and high fever. If a patient on NSAIDs develops these symptoms, the physician will probably order a spinal
tap to evaluate the spinal fluid to determine if there is an infection
before prescribing treatment. This complication is rare.

Fluid retention. NSAIDs are likely to worsen edema in patients
with swelling, especially in the ankles. This complication is more
likely to be seen in patients who have low albumin levels in their
blood due to kidney disease.

Rare complications. Although it is extremely rare, some patients may develop other serious complications from an NSAID,
including skin rashes, suppression of the bone marrow, and other
problems. Contact your physician immediately if you break out
into a rash or notice any other physical change. Patients on these
drugs should have their blood counts checked periodically, which
should be done for most SLE patients anyway.

ANTIMALARIAL DRUGS

Drugs used for the treatment of malaria have been found to be extremely effective in treating rashes related to SLE, including discoid lupus as well as mouth ulcers, arthritis, and other symptoms. The antimalarial medications include hydroxychlorquine (Plaquenil) and chloroquine (Aralen, Quinacrine, and Atabrine). The exact mechanism of action of these drugs in SLE is unknown, although they appear to have anti-inflammatory and immunosuppressive properties.

Antimalarial drugs appear to be well tolerated by SLE patients and have relatively few side effects. Studies show that patients on antimalarial drugs appear to have fewer flares than those not taking these medications.

Antimalarial drugs are long acting; it may take weeks or months for the patient to show any signs of improvement. Usually, skin rashes will respond to these drugs before joint pain or other arthritic symptoms will.

✎ SIDE EFFECTS

Vision impairment. Antimalarials can cause damage to the eyes, particularly to the retina, called *retinopathy*. Any patient starting on this course of treatment should be seen by an ophthalmologist for a baseline examination and then examined periodically thereafter (usually every 3 to 6 months). The patient should watch out for a change in the ability to see red as well as light flashes or streaks. Because these problems can go unnoticed, frequent eye exams are essential.

Some ophthalmologists may give their patients a red piece of paper to check monthly for change in color vision. Patients are instructed to call their doctors if the paper appears to be a different color (darker or lighter). In addition, patients may be given an Amsler grid (which looks like a piece of graph paper), which may help them to detect loss of peripheral vision. Patients should contact their doctors if they notice any change in their vision.

Antimalarial retinopathy can be worsened by exposure to sun; therefore, patients should wear UV-protective sunglasses.

Increased photosensitivity. Some patients on antimalarials can get hyperpigmentation from the sun, that is, exposure to the sun can give their skin a darker, grayish pigmentation. Rarely, their hair may become bleached. Needless to say, SLE patients in general and patients on antimalarials in particular should avoid exposure to sun.

Hair loss. Some women on antimalarials report mild hair loss. However, it is difficult to distinguish this from the normal hair loss that may occur in SLE.

Peripheral neuropathy. Some patients may develop nerve damage with no symptoms initially, but that will become apparent during a physical exam by the doctor. Reflexes of patients on these drugs should be monitored by the physician. Muscle weakness could also be a danger sign, although other causes would need to be ruled out.

Rare complications. Patients with an enzyme deficiency in their red blood cells, called G-6-PD deficiency, may develop severe hemolytic anemia and should be closely monitored with CBCs. In other extremely rare cases, these medications can result in suppression of the bone marrow, so patients on these drugs need to have their blood counts checked routinely.

CORTICOSTEROIDS

Patients with symptoms that do not improve or are not expected to respond to NSAIDs or antimalarials may be put on corticosteroids, a class of drugs related to cortisone, which is one of the hormones produced by the adrenal gland. Although cortisone is normally present in the body, the synthetic versions, which are often given in much higher doses than the body produces, are potent therapeutic agents. (Although they may share some common characteristics, corticosteroids are quite different from anabolic steroids, substances that are abused by body builders, or sex hormones, which are also steroidal compounds.)

Corticosteroids may be used in a variety of ways: as a topical cream or ointment for skin rashes; injected into the joints for arthritis; taken orally or given as an intravenous (IV) or intramuscular injection.

Women with symptoms such as extreme fatigue, severe arthritis, pleuritis, pericarditis, uncontrolled fever, or kidney disease may be put on an oral dose of a corticosteroid, such as prednisone, prednisolone, or methylprednisolone (Medrol).

Oral steroids are typically taken once daily, usually in the morning, although in severe cases, several doses per day may be given for a limited time. However, some physicians may prescribe an alternate-day steroid regimen, which requires taking a higher dose every other day. Some studies suggest that the alternate-day method may be just as effective as the daily method but have less side effects.

Although corticosteroids have many potentially dangerous side effects, they are truly wonderful drugs and often give new life to SLE patients. They are highly effective in reducing inflammation, relieving muscle and joint pain and fatigue, and suppressing the immune system. These drugs are particularly useful in controlling major organ involvement of SLE including kidney disease and thrombocytopenia.

In moderate doses, SLE patients fare well on corticosteroids and seem to tolerate these drugs better than patients who must take them for other ailments. The goal, however, should be to get down to the lowest possible dose that can safely control the activity of the disease. The dose for each patient is highly individual. Therefore, when a patient is put on steroids, she must work closely with her physician to determine what dose works best for her. The physician relies on her feedback to help determine the appropriate and safest dose.

Many physicians occasionally give patients some discretion regarding the use of steroids. If a doctor knows a patient well and respects her judgment, he or she will at times allow her to modestly increase her dose of steroids on her own when she is in pain. However, if a patient finds that she is increasing her dose more than once or twice a month, she should call her doctor for an alternative treatment plan. Because steroids work so fast and so well, there is tendency on the part of some patients to overuse them: *Do not exceed your prescribed dose without consulting with your physician.* The injudicious use of steroids can, in many cases, pose even more serious problems than SLE.

During times of serious illness, corticosteroids may be administered intravenously, because they can be given in higher doses and are better absorbed by the body. When stabilized, the patient is switched to an oral dose of steroids.

Steroids can never be discontinued abruptly; they must be tapered off gradually. *You cannot allow your supply of steroids to run out or accidentally skip a few days without risking serious consequences*, such as a sudden flare or a condition called *adrenal insufficiency*. In the latter case, the pituitary gland, which stimulates the adrenal gland to produce cortisone, may have shut down in response to the synthetic cortisone. The adrenal gland itself may also be atrophied as a result. Thus, when the synthetic cortisone is suddenly taken away, the pituitary gland may fail to stimulate the adrenal gland, or it may be unable to respond, either of which can result in severe problems for the patient. Symptoms of adrenal insufficiency may be vague and include fatigue, fever, weight loss, anorexia, gastrointestinal discomfort, and, less commonly, low blood pressure and dizziness upon standing. To avoid the risk of adrenal insufficiency, if a patient has been on more than 10 milligrams of prednisone or its equivalent for a prolonged period of time within the past year, she may require a higher "stress dose" of steroids prior to a physically stressful event, such as labor and delivery, surgery, or after severe trauma such as a car accident. I advise patients who may require stress-dose steroids to wear a medic alert bracelet.

Because of these risks, tapering a patient off steroids or even reducing the dose must be done very carefully. Very often, during the tapering period, patients experience what appears to be a flare each time their dose of steroid is reduced—they develop joint and muscle pain, fever, and fatigue. This is often not a real flare, rather it is the body reacting to missing the larger dose. To avoid severe problems, the dose should be decreased very gradually over a period of time. Usually, within 3 to 5 days, the patient will feel better and will be ready for another reduction in the dose of steroid. (If not, they could be experiencing a flare.) The doctor will stop cutting the drug when the patient reaches the lowest dose at which she remains symptom-free. Some patients may be able to live steroid-free except for periods of active disease; others may need to be maintained on a low dose chronically.

People who are undergoing the tapering process require a lot of support and encouragement from their physicians, families, and friends. It's especially important for them to remember that the discomfort is temporary, and in most cases, they will be feeling well within a short period of time.

⤴ SIDE EFFECTS

Susceptibility to infection. Steroids suppress the immune system, which can leave the body more vulnerable to certain infections, including pneumonia, urinary infections, and vaginal yeast infections. Certain infections, such as shingles (reactivated chicken pox) and TB, can be reactivated when a patient is on steroids (or any other immunosuppressive drug). Therefore, it's advisable to perform a PPD or Mantoux skin test to check for previous TB exposure prior to putting a patient on a high dose of steroids. (In this test, a small injection of a protein from the TB bacillus is placed under the skin. If after twenty-four to forty-eight hours the patient develops a raised bump on the skin, it could indicate previous TB exposure.) Once the patient is on steroids, it is very difficult to get an accurate test for TB. If the skin test is positive or the patient has a prior history of TB, the physician may also want to do a chest X ray to assess for active disease. In some cases, the physician may want to put the patient on a prophylactic antituberculous regimen prior to or concomitant with giving steroids to prevent reactivation of the infection.

Obesity. Steroids cause an increase in appetite, which can result in excess weight gain. In addition, these drugs actually alter the way fat is deposited in the body, resulting in a round or moon face and a wide, thick trunk. In some cases, a fat deposit known as a "buffalo hump" may appear on the upper back.

High blood pressure. Steroids can cause an increase in blood pressure due partly to salt and fluid retention.

Diabetes. There is an added risk of developing diabetes on high doses of steroids.

Excess hair growth. Patients on steroids may experience an excess growth of body hair, especially on the face.

Thin skin. Topical or systemic steroids can cause the epidermis or outer layer of skin to thin, creating a papery, wrinkled appearance. In the case of topical steroids, a lightening of the skin color may be the first sign of thinning. If the steroids are discontinued, much of this damage can be reversed.

Steroids can also cause stretch marks (striae) in areas of sudden weight gain, especially on the abdomen and thighs. Unlike normal stretch marks, these are a more noticeable lavender and reddish color and improve very slowly, if at all, with weight loss. (This is one of the reasons why it's so important to try to maintain normal weight.)

Muscle weakness. Patients on steroids may experience muscle weakness, especially in the large muscles of the leg. Typically, they may feel weak when walking up a flight of stairs or standing up from a seated position.

Psychiatric problems. Steroids can cause dramatic psychiatric changes, including depression, mania, sleeplessness, and psychosis. (The latter usually only occurs at very high doses.)

Premature osteoporosis. Women on chronic steroids are at greater risk of developing thin or brittle bones, which can result in bone fractures (three times the rate of normal) and loss of height. One steroid preparation called deflazacort, widely used in Europe but not yet available in the United States, is believed to be bone sparing compared to the other preparations used here. If it becomes available in the United States, hopefully some of these bone loss problems can be avoided.

Increased blood lipids. Steroids can cause a significant increase in blood cholesterol, possibly putting the patient at greater risk of developing coronary artery disease if cholesterol is elevated chronically.

Poor wound healing. Steroids can prevent wounds from healing quickly. If a patient on a high dose of steroids undergoes surgery, the surgeon may choose to leave the stitches in longer, allowing for more time to heal.

IMMUNOSUPPRESSIVE DRUGS

The immunosuppressive drugs azathioprine (Imuran) and cyclophosphamide (Cytoxan) were initially used in chemotherapy for cancer patients. They are strong medicine, so strong in fact that they are used to treat SLE only when absolutely necessary. Usually, this class of drug is reserved for patients with major organ involvement, severe muscle inflammation, or intractable arthritis. A patient may be treated with immunosuppressive therapy in conjunction with steroids, permitting the use of a lower dose of steroids, or when being tapered off steroids to avoid a major flare.

Immunosuppressive drugs work by killing rapidly dividing cells; they are effective against tumor cells, lymphocytes, and other white blood cells in the immune system. They also have complex effects on the inflammatory process.

Imuran is usually taken orally daily. Cytoxan may be given

orally daily or intravenously. Since oral Cytoxan appears to increase the risk of developing bladder cancer, IV Cytoxan is the preferred method since it can be given with lots of fluid, which reduces the risk of bladder damage. IV Cytoxan may be administered in the hospital, in the doctor's office, or by a home infusion service. A drug called mesna (Mesnex) may be given to reduce the risk of developing bladder hemorrhage and subsequent cancer.

Similar to chemotherapy for cancer, IV Cytoxan is given in courses. It may be given monthly for up to three to six months and then usually decreased to every three months. Within ten days after treatment, there is usually a decrease in the white blood cell count, showing a dramatic decline in immune activity. It could take several weeks before the patient shows clinical improvement in symptoms and evidence of disease activity.

Because these drugs have such a powerful effect on the immune system, any patient who has been sexually active within the past ten years should be tested for HIV before undergoing immunosuppressive therapy. Some of the symptoms of AIDS are similar to SLE, and if an already immunocompromised AIDS patient were to receive immunosuppressive therapy, it could be devastating.

❧ SIDE EFFECTS

Extreme nausea. Patients on IV Cytoxan in particular may experience extreme nausea during treatment. There are now some excellent antiemetic drugs, such as ondansetron (Zofran),which can help virtually eliminate nausea and vomiting.

Hair loss. Similar to chemotherapy patients, SLE patients on immunosuppressive drugs often lose their hair as a result of treatment. However, it will grow back, though the texture and the color may be significantly different for some time.

Increased risk of infection. The purpose of immunosuppressive therapy is to reduce the activity of the immune system. However, in the process, it may leave the body vulnerable to infections, such as shingles, fungal infections, TB, and other forms of pneumonia.

Suppression of bone marrow. Immunosuppressive drugs can result in severe anemia (low levels of red blood cells) and a dangerous decline in white blood cells and platelets, placing the patient at risk of infection and bleeding. It is critical for patients on these drugs to have their blood counts and blood chemistries monitored frequently.

Premature menopause and infertility. Patients on Cytoxan may stop menstruating or undergo premature menopause. In cancer patients, physicians believe that suppressing ovulation with birth control pills during treatment may help preserve ovarian function. The use of birth control pills in lupus is controversial, however, because many physicians believe that estrogen can trigger a flare. The younger a woman is during treatment and the shorter the duration of treatment, the less likely that this problem will develop.

Blood in urine. Patients on oral Cytoxan may develop blood in the urine, a sign of bladder irritation that could lead to cancer. These patients should contact their doctor immediately. Urinalysis should be monitored periodically for blood.

Late malignancies. There is an ongoing controversy as to whether patients who have been treated with immunosuppressive drugs are at an increased risk for malignancy (usually lymphoma, a tumor of the lymph tissues) years after treatment. Some researchers feel that the cases reported were a coincidence, some blame a chronically overactive immune system—the disease itself—as causing the problem, but others place the blame on the immunosuppressive drugs. We don't have an answer yet, but this is another reason why these drugs are reserved for patients with severe disease or for those who are unresponsive to milder therapies.

EXPERIMENTAL THERAPIES

Before I describe some of the new treatments that are being studied for lupus, I want to strongly caution patients about seeking out unconventional or unproven therapies. As of yet, there is no cure or panacea for lupus. If anyone tells you that there is, he or she is lying. Unfortunately, patients with chronic illnesses such as lupus or arthritis are often preyed upon by unscrupulous people who make all sorts of promises, demand high payment, and deliver nothing. In some cases, their treatments may be completely useless; in others, they may be downright dangerous, especially if a patient gets sicker because she discontinued or rejected a proven treatment for one that is ineffective. Although most of these charlatans are not physicians, some may be. (Being an M.D. does not automatically mean that someone is acting in a moral or ethical way.) There are also many alternative health practitioners who may claim and even believe that they have found the "cure." They haven't. Lupus is an extremely complex disorder involving the equally complex immune system. As we have seen with AIDS, the mechanisms of the immune system are very complicated. There are no quick fixes or easy solutions. Dabbling in experimental and unproven treatments could hurt both your pocketbook and your health.

There are, however, some promising legitimate treatments on the horizon that one day may become accepted medical practice. Before any procedure can be considered an accepted form of treatment in the United States, it must be carefully evaluated in clinical studies performed at an academic medical center or research institution. The physicians or researchers conducting the investigation are subject to close scrutiny by an institutional review board to ensure that the study is being performed with high scientific and ethical standards and that the study will yield information that will benefit all patients. Study patients sign a statement of informed consent prior to the study in which they are made aware of the risks and benefits of this particular treatment, especially if there is a chance that they may be given a placebo (a sugar pill instead of the study treatment) instead of the available conventional therapies.

I want to caution patients in particular about experimental treatments being offered outside of the United States. Many countries do not have the same safeguards to protect patients, and you could be putting yourself at great risk if you try an experimental treatment without adequate supervision or follow-up.

There are two kinds of patients who may wish to consider participating in a study of experimental therapy. The first are patients who have not been helped by conventional treatments and may want to try a different approach. These patients are usually quite sick and are so desperate for help that they are willing to take the risk of trying an experimental therapy. The second are patients who have very mild symptoms, so mild, in fact, that it's not particularly urgent to start them on proven remedies. If you are being treated for your lupus symptoms with conventional therapies and are doing well, I don't advise trying an experimental therapy. You have little to gain and a lot to lose if it doesn't work.

If you are interested in participating in clinical studies, contact the division of rheumatology or immunology at your local hospital or medical school or the local chapters of the Lupus Foundation or the Arthritis Foundation to make certain that the investigators are well qualified to perform the study. Call the National Institutes of Health in Bethesda, Maryland (see Resources), to find out about research being done in your area.

Experimental treatments are not usually covered by insurance and should be paid for by the hospital or institution conducting the study. The treatment and related follow-up should be free. You may be required to pay for routine care and tests. However, if you're asked to fork out a lot of money to participate in an experimental procedure, don't do it.

Many of the accepted treatments we use today were once regarded as experimental therapies, and we owe a debt of gratitude to the patients who took part in earlier clinical studies. In the future, I hope that there will be more carefully controlled studies so that we can find new and more effective therapies.

Following is a list of some of the most interesting new treatments that may one day become part of mainstream therapy.

∽ IV GAMMA-GLOBULIN. Gamma-globulin is a purified blood product that consists of the pooled antibodies from literally thousands of donors. In this procedure, gamma-globulin is given intravenously to lupus patients. It has been successfully used to treat thrombocytopenia and some forms of vasculitis. Why would lupus patients, who produce too much antibody to begin with, benefit from extra antibodies? Researchers speculate that when introduced into the body of lupus patients, the antibodies from other patients may somehow turn off cells in the immune system, specifically the B cells, that trigger the production of too much antibody. Another possible explanation revolves around the relationship between antigens, substances that the body regards as foreign and the antibodies it produces to protect itself against these unwanted invaders. Antigens and antibodies come together to form immune complexes. In the case of SLE, these immune complexes go on to attack the body's own tissues. However, if you add additional foreign antibodies into the mix through IV gamma-globulin, it may be possible to change the size of the immune complexes in such a way that they can't lodge in sensitive tissues and cause damage. This treatment is not used very often because it is very expensive but may prove to be useful in severe cases.

☘ PLASMAPHERESIS. In this procedure, plasma from the patient's blood is withdrawn and the immunoglobulin (antibodies) removed. The plasma minus the immune complexes is returned to the patient. This procedure is very expensive and has not yielded consistent results, except in some cases of vasculitis. Although it has generally fallen out of favor, it is still sometimes tried for desperately ill patients when all else has failed.

☘ PLASMAPHERESIS COMBINED WITH IV CYTOXAN. This procedure, which is being evaluated in an international study, combines plasmapheresis with IV high doses of the immunosuppressive drug Cytoxan. The theory behind this combined therapy is appealing: Researchers speculate that when the immune complexes are removed from the plasma, the B cells are stimulated to produce more antibody. The Cytoxan, in turn, will destroy the rapidly proliferating B cells, thus reducing the formation of new antibodies. So far, preliminary data are good, but it will take a few years before we know if this treatment is effective.

☘ METHOTREXATE. This drug, used in chemotherapy for cancer patients, is also an approved treatment for patients with rheumatoid arthritis and psoriasis. Preliminary studies show promise for patients with lupus, particularly those with joint involvement. However, it can cause liver damage, and patients on this drug must be closely monitored.

☘ HORMONAL THERAPY. Studies of lupus patients have shown that both men and women with lupus appear to metabolize or break down the female hormone estrogen differently than other people. Other studies have shown that hormones in general appear to have an effect on the immune system; generally, estrogen and possibly prolactin (a pituitary hormone) have some immune-stimulating effects, but progesterone and testosterone seem to suppress it. Some researchers are attempting to suppress the overactive immune system typical of lupus by giving patients androgens, or male hormones. So far, a form of androgen (Danazol) has been effective for immune thrombocytopenia and a handful of other immune disorders. Treatment of lupus with androgens has been inconsistent to date. Preliminary studies show bromocryptine (which suppresses prolactin) and leuprolide (which suppresses ovarian function) may have immunosuppressant effects in lupus. Clearly, more studies are needed to see if hormonal manipulations could be helpful in lupus.

❧ MONOCLONAL ANTIBODY THERAPY. Conventional immunosuppressive treatment for lupus dampens the entire immune system; it suppresses good cells as well as bad cells, leaving the patient vulnerable to infection. In monoclonal antibody therapy, researchers are trying to develop specific antibodies to knock out the cells that are involved in the overproduction of autoantibodies. In some studies, researchers have targeted the CD4 lymphocyte (T-helper cell), which is believed to be involved in promoting B-cell overactivity in lupus. We are still in the earliest stages in the research to design more sophisticated and specific treatments that target the key lymphocytes that are out of balance in lupus. In years to come, we will hear more about these innovative treatments.

❧ OMEGA-3 FATTY ACID (FISH OIL). Omega-3 refers to two types of polyunsaturated fatty acids: docosahexaenoic acid and eicosapentaenoic acid. Omega-3's are found primarily in marine plant life called *phytoplankton* and on land in flaxseed. Fish such as salmon, cod, halibut, albacore tuna, bass, sardines, and mackerel, which feed on omega-3-rich plants, are primary sources of omega-3 for humans. Omega-3 fatty acids have an anti-inflammatory effect by altering the way substances called *prostaglandins* are made in the body. Several studies have shown that rheumatoid arthritis patients have experienced a significant reduction in symptoms after taking omega-3 fatty acid supplements. In fact, according to a recent study, patients fared as well on a high dose of fish oil capsules as they did on NSAIDs. In studies in mice but not patients with lupus, some benefit has been noted. More study is needed to determine whether fish oil capsules would offer lupus patients relief from joint aches and pains. Fish oil may possibly offer an additional benefit to some women with SLE: Omega-3 fatty acid is also a blood thinner, which could help prevent clotting in women with antiphospholipid antibodies. A word of caution: Do not take fish oil supplements on your own, especially if you already take aspirin or other blood-thinning medications, without consulting your doctor.

❧ COMBINATION IMMUNOSUPPRESSIVE THERAPY. Researchers are trying various combinations of immunosuppressive drugs to treat lupus, such as Cyclosporine and Imuran. These drugs are very powerful and can cause dangerous side effects, for example, Cyclosporine can be toxic to the kidneys. Therefore, these patients should be closely monitored.

❧ TOTAL LYMPH NODE IRRADIATION. Irradiation of the thymus, spleen, and major lymph node groups done repeatedly has a long-lasting immunosuppressive effect, notably, a decline in CD4 T-helper cells, which has a profound effect on the immune system. The risk of this treatment is similar to that of immunosuppressive drug regimens (see p. 73).

CHAPTER 5

Managing Your Health

When you have a chronic disease such as SLE, your doctor can help you manage your symptoms and is there to care for you if you get sick, but you are the only one who can maintain your health on a daily basis. Therefore, it is critical for you to learn how to manage and preserve your own health.

Although you may not be able to cure your lupus, in some cases, you may be able to control flares by avoiding known *triggers*, things that can exacerbate your lupus. You may also help to prevent other medical problems that can exacerbate your symptoms. In addition, an alert patient may be able to catch small problems early on before they develop into bigger ones. Finally, if you maintain as high a level of health and fitness as you can when you are well, you will be in a stronger position to deal with the times when you may get sick.

AVOIDING INFECTION

Lupus patients need to be concerned about avoiding infection for several reasons. First, lupus patients may be more prone to contracting certain infections due to the effect of immunosuppressive drugs they are taking for SLE, such as prednisone or aza-thathioprine. Second, despite the fact that lupus patients have overactive immune systems, in many cases, they are actually more vulnerable to contracting certain infections than other people, and when they do get sick, it may be more severe. Finally, in some patients, infections can trigger flares. Therefore, the primary goal should be to stay as healthy and illness-free as possible.

Lupus patients should be immunized against pneumococcal pneumonia, a type of bacterial pneumonia to which lupus patients are particularly vulnerable. In addition, lupus patients are advised to receive a flu shot every fall.

Although it can be difficult to avoid contracting colds and viruses, there are some steps that you can take to minimize your risk. If you are taking an immunosuppressive medication, try to avoid coming in contact with contagious people. This doesn't mean that you have to live in a glass bubble; however, it means taking certain commonsense precautions against getting sick. For example, avoid crowded, stuffy public places during the height of flu season, and let friends and relatives know that you would prefer canceling an appointment to being exposed to a contagious cold or viral infection. Even if you're not immunosuppressed, it makes good sense to practice good hygiene: Wash your hands after going to the bathroom and before cooking or touching your mouth and nose. If you have a young child or take care of sick people, be especially vigilant about hand washing. Avoid sharing towels with other people; keep your towel separate and don't share drinking glasses or utensils with other people.

People with suppressed immune systems are also more prone to contract food poisoning, notably salmonella and *Escherichia coli* bacteria. Be especially careful about handling eggs and raw poultry, major sources of salmonella in the United States. Wash your hands very well with soap and hot water after touching raw eggs or chicken. Wash any utensils and surfaces that have come in contact with raw eggs or chicken very carefully with hot water and detergent. Cook chicken and eggs very well before eating; rare chicken or wet, runny eggs are not safe. In addition, be aware that rare or undercooked meat of any kind could be tainted with *E. coli* bacteria; do not eat raw or undercooked meat. If you eat out, do not order rare meat, especially hamburger, which because of the way it's processed is more prone to be tainted with *E. coli*.

KNOW THE SIGNS OF TROUBLE

Your doctor should be alerted about any change in symptoms or worsening of your disease as soon as possible. However, a lupus patient should know exactly what symptoms are so serious that you need to see your doctor right away or go to an emergency room. The following symptoms are serious enough to warrant immediate medical attention.

1. If you always have a fever and you're taking only anti-inflammatory medication, a fever is normal for you. However, if you develop a new fever, a much higher fever, or any fever at all while taking an immunosuppressive medication, you need to call your doctor immediately. It could be a sign of infection or a lupus flare.

2. If you have any seizures, call your doctor. This is a manifestation of CNS disease and a medical emergency.

3. If you have a severe headache with neck stiffness and fever, you could have developed meningitis, a brain infection. Contact your doctor as this is a medical emergency.

4. If you feel any chest pain, call your doctor. It could be pericarditis or pleuritis and should be treated promptly.

5. If you feel any swelling or pain in your leg (especially around the calf), call your doctor. It could be a sign of a blood clot.

6. If you have severe abdominal pain, call your doctor. It could be an ulcer from medication (if you are taking NSAIDs), vasculitis of the gastrointestinal tract, or even appendicitis.

7. If you have any blood in the stool, vomit blood, or have dark black stool, call your doctor. It could be a sign of intestinal bleeding from an ulcer.

8. If you experience any confusion or mood changes, call your doctor. It could be a sign of CNS disease or a reaction to steroids.

9. If you have bleeding or excessive bruising anywhere on your body, call your doctor. It could be a sign of a dropping platelet count. You doctor needs to know about this at once.

There are symptoms that may not be life-threatening but may indicate that you are heading in the wrong direction and may need to change treatment. If you experience any of these symptoms, call your doctor to schedule an appointment.

1. Increased rash.
2. Increased or new hair loss.
3. Increased joint pain.
4. Foamy urine.
5. Sores or ulcers in your mouth.

YOUR GENERAL HEALTH

In addition to monitoring your lupus symptoms, you also need to maintain your overall health. Every woman with lupus should have an annual physical in which her primary care physician examines her carefully and tracks her progress. Like other women, women with lupus should have mammograms: a baseline after age thirty-five, every other year after age forty, and annually after age fifty. (If you have a mother or sister with breast cancer, your physician may recommend an earlier baseline.) Women with lupus, especially those on steroids, need to have their blood lipid levels (cholesterol and triglycerides) periodically monitored before menopause and monitored annually after menopause when the risk for developing heart disease rises significantly for women in general and for women with SLE in particular. (Cholesterol should be 230 milligrams per deciliter or below; triglycerides should not exceed 190 milligrams per deciliter.) In addition, women with lupus, especially those who are postmenopausal or have been on high doses of steroids, may need to have a bone density assessment for osteoporosis.

In addition, women with SLE may have particular health problems that require visits to other specialists or special precautions that they must take on their own.

GYNECOLOGIC CARE

A woman with SLE should have an annual internal examination performed by a gynecologist or a primary care physician. Studies show that women with lupus have a higher rate of abnormal Pap tests than other women because they are more likely to develop vaginal warts or herpes due to immunosuppressive drugs or to have low-grade infections. If untreated or chronic, these problems could increase the risk of cancer.

Women on steroids may experience menstrual abnormalities, such as bleeding in between periods or irregular periods, which return to normal when the drug is discontinued. However, women taking Cytoxan may develop premature menopause, especially if they are over thirty-five.

VAGINAL DRYNESS

Vaginal dryness due to a lack of vaginal secretions, which may be caused by Sjogren's syndrome, certain medications, or menopause, is a common problem for women with SLE. Commercially sold lubricants, such as Replens and K-Y Jelly, can help replace the lost moisture. It is especially important to use a lubricant prior to sexual intercourse. (Do not use petroleum jelly; it can actually promote infection by providing a favorable growth environment for yeast and bacteria.) Due to vaginal dryness, patients who use tampons may be at greater risk of tearing vaginal tissue, which can increase the risk of toxic shock syndrome. Therefore, these patients should be very careful about using a personal lubricant before inserting the tampon. If you are very dry, use sanitary pads instead.

YEAST INFECTIONS

Due to suppressed immunity, women with SLE are also more prone to contract a yeast infection, which is characterized by vaginal itching and a thick, white discharge. At least one study showed that women who eat an 8-ounce container of yogurt daily with active live cultures of the bacterium *Lactobacillus acidophilus* can help prevent the onset of yeast infections. (Read the label carefully. Many brands of yogurt, especially the whipped or swiss style, do not contain active cultures.) In addition, 500 milligrams of vitamin C daily may decrease the risk of vaginal yeast and bladder infections. Also, avoid wearing tight pants or nylon underwear, which don't allow for adequate ventilation. (Yeast thrive in a moist, warm environment.)

URINARY TRACT INFECTIONS

Women with lupus should be aware of the fact that they can easily be misdiagnosed as having a urinary tract infection (UTI) when in fact they are developing new kidney disease. For example, if a young woman who is running a high fever and feels very sick goes to an emergency room, the doctor on call will undoubtedly take a urine sample. If the urine reveals the presence of red and white blood cells, the doctor will assume that the woman has a UTI, which is quite common in young women, and may not culture the urine, that is, check it for bacterial growth. In fact, he or she will probably prescribe an antibiotic, often ampicillin or a sulfa-based drug, both of which may cause bad reactions in some women with SLE. The patient may take the drug and get even sicker. Hopefully, if a woman is being treated by her usual doctor, he or she will exercise proper caution with the diagnosis and treatment of a UTI. Women with lupus should not accept a diagnosis of UTI without a culture; the symptoms for UTI and kidney disease are too similar, and further testing is required. However, if the symptoms are severe, it may be necessary to begin treating the infection pending the culture result.

BIRTH CONTROL

Because most of the women diagnosed with SLE are in their childbearing years, birth control is an important issue—it is also a controversial one. The two most convenient methods of birth control, the birth control pill and the intrauterine device (IUD) have been considered off-limits for women with SLE. The IUD, which is inserted into the cervix, can promote infection. Because women with SLE are already more prone to certain infections, they should steer clear of this method of contraception. The birth control pill, containing estrogen and/or progesterone, is the most popular method of contraception in the world. Yet, women with SLE are routinely advised not to use it, because the handful of studies that have been conducted suggest that estrogen may cause flares. Other hormonal forms of contraception such as Norplant, a long-acting progesterone capsule that is implanted under the skin, has not been studied in women with lupus.

On what do we base our recommendations? There is strong evidence that women with antiphospholipid antibodies should steer clear of the Pill because estrogen can promote blood clots, and the Pill has been associated with severe problems in these patients. However, there have not been enough studies on SLE women without antiphospholipid antibodies to know for sure whether the Pill or Norplant are harmful for these women. It's possible that the newer, low-dose estrogen pill or the progesterone-only pill may be safe for women with mild disease who would be good candidates for the Pill under other circumstances (that is, they don't smoke, do not have a family history of breast cancer, and are not hypertensive). It just may be that given the choice of using the Pill or not using contraception, the Pill may be safer than an unplanned pregnancy. Unfortunately, we just don't know enough to help patients make an intelligent choice. There is growing interest in answering these questions, and several studies are underway that may shed some light.

Due to the lack of information, most women with SLE should use barrier method contraception such as the diaphragm or male condom in combination with spermicidal foam. However, if a woman with mild disease is on the Pill and having no trouble, she does not have to stop, especially if she has made it clear that she is unwilling to use other contraceptive methods.

SEXUALLY TRANSMITTED DISEASES

Whatever method you choose for birth control, it is very important that your partner use a condom. Every sexually active woman today needs to be concerned about contracting HIV, however, some women with SLE may be at somewhat higher risk. Studies show that women with vaginal ulcers are at substantially greater risk of contracting HIV and other venereal diseases from their partners. Because you may have vaginal ulcers and not even know it, it is even more critical that you give yourself the protection you need. You may have heard about a new female condom that is currently on the market. It does not appear to be as reliable a contraceptive as other methods but may help to prevent against sexually transmitted diseases.

You also need to protect yourself against other common sexually transmitted diseases: herpes, gonorrhea, and syphilis. Herpes simplex virus type 2 is characterized by tiny but painful ulcers in the vaginal and rectal area and sometimes the mouth. When the disease is active, the person may experience flulike symptoms for a few days. After the initial herpes attack, the signs and symptoms of the virus lay dormant, ready to strike at any time. Although women with lupus are not more prone to contract herpes, the herpes virus may be reactivated when they are put on immunosuppressive drugs. A woman with lupus should avoid getting herpes in the first place by asking her partner to use condoms; if she has a history of herpes, she should have her partner wear condoms to protect him from contracting this virus.

Women with lupus, especially those with low complement levels, are more prone to develop a particularly severe form of gonorrhea called *disseminated gonorrhea*, in which the infection enters the bloodstream and can cause fever and arthritic symptoms. If contracted, this type of gonorrhea may go undiagnosed for some time because it so closely resembles a lupus flare. Another sexually transmitted disease, syphilis, also resembles lupus in many ways; in fact, about 20 percent of all women with lupus have a false-positive blood test for syphilis. A physician may not be able to distinguish syphilis from lupus, at least in the earliest stages. To avoid diagnostic confusion, your best bet is to avoid contracting these diseases. If you have been married for years or in a long-term stable monogamous relationship, these issues may be of less concern. A discussion with your gynecologist may be helpful.

AGING-RELATED CONCERNS

As women with lupus live longer, other gynecological questions are beginning to emerge. For example, we know that post-menopausal women in general and women who have had steroid treatment in particular are at greater risk of developing osteoporosis, a potentially debilitating disease characterized by the thinning of the bones, which can result in fractures, usually of the hip or vertebrae. In fact, complications from osteoporosis are a leading cause of death among older women. The number one cause of death among women past age sixty is heart disease, another problem that women with SLE are prone to develop after menopause.

Several studies performed on postmenopausal women without lupus suggest that hormonal replacement therapy may help prevent both osteoporosis and heart disease. Obviously, it would be a boon for SLE women if they could safely take hormonal replacement therapy, particularly those who had been on steroids and are at particularly high risk of losing bone density or developing atherosclerosis, later in life. However, because of the adverse experiences with early studies of high-dose estrogen birth control pills, there have been few studies on hormone replacement therapy and lupus. In a recent study in England of postmenopausal SLE patients with relatively mild and stable disease, the women were able to take estrogen safely. Experience has been very limited, and many more studies need to be done before we can confidently prescribe hormone replacement therapy to women with lupus.

It is very clear, however, that women with antiphospholipid antibodies should not take hormones in any form because of the increased risk of blood clotting.

SKIN CARE

About 40 to 60 percent of all SLE patients are photosensitive, that is, UV light from the sun and other sources actually worsens their symptoms. Photosensitivity can develop at any point in lupus—even if you're not photosensitive now, you may be later. Many patients with mild disease return from vacations with bad flares, all because they allowed themselves to bask in the sun. It is advisable for all SLE patients to avoid exposure to sun. In fact, even if patients don't have lupus but have a close relative with lupus, they should also limit sun exposure. Given the fact that we now know that sun exposure can increase the risk of developing skin cancer and can cause premature aging (a problem that appears to have been aggravated by the thinning of the ozone layer), this advice is not particularly radical.

SUNSCREEN PROTECTION

Limiting exposure to the sun doesn't mean that you have to stay indoors during daylight hours with the blinds drawn. It does mean that you have to exercise certain precautions. Lupus patients should try to avoid prolonged outdoor activities between the hours of 10 A.M. and 3 P.M. When you do go out, you should wear a sunscreen with a SPF (sun protection factor) of 15 or higher on exposed areas. (The SPF rating means that you can stay out in the sun that many times longer with the sunscreen protection on, without burning, than without it.) Reapply the sunscreen after swimming or excessive sweating.

Be sure to check that the sunscreen protects against both UVB and UVA rays. Some only protect against UVB or offer minimal UVA protection—you need protection against both. UVB rays are responsible for burning, wrinkling, and causing skin injury that can result in cancer. They can also aggravate lupus. UVA, the so-called tanning rays, were once believed to be safe, but we now know that they can also cause the kind of skin damage that can trigger a lupus flare.

Before using a sunscreen product, read the label carefully. Check with your dermatologist if you're not sure about the ingredients. Although formulas for sunscreens vary, in general, PABA (*para*-aminobenzoic acid) a common ingredient, absorbs only UVB; benzophenones and anthranilates absorb both UVA and UVB. Shade UVA Guard and Photoplex are two sunscreens that protect against both UVA and UVB. People with sensitive skin may be allergic to PABA or other chemicals in sunscreens. If you break out in a rash or develop an irritation after using a brand, discontinue using it, and check with your doctor for alternative recommendations.

Some dermatologists recommend that you test any new skin product for a potential allergic reaction before using it. Smear the product on a quarter-size area of skin in the evening and check the area for irritation the next morning. However, some allergic reactions may not be triggered until your treated skin is exposed to the sun, so this test is not foolproof.

Sunscreen is not just for the summer; UV light can be reflected by snow and even concrete. UV light can even filter through clouds, so use sun protection all year, even on days that are not sunny. Always use sunscreen at the beach, even if you're sitting under an umbrella, because UV light is reflected off of sand. UVA light is not filtered out by glass; therefore, you can't sunbathe safely in a glass-enclosed room or at a glass-topped swimming pool. In addition, if you work near a window either at home or at the office, be sure to keep the shades down at least during the peak sun hours, and don't forget to wear sunscreen. UV-filtering glass or film can be used in automobiles for added protection.

Many cosmetics today include UV protection. If you wear makeup, you might as well use one that offers this added benefit. A sun hat also offers additional protection but is not a replacement for sunscreen.

PROTECTIVE CLOTHING

If you're outdoors a great deal, wear protective clothing; don't walk around in a bathing suit or a tank top. Dark clothing with a heavy weave offers the best sun protection; however, it is not very comfortable in the warm months. A summer-weight dry T-shirt naturally offers an SPF of 5 to 7, which may not be enough for someone who is photosensitive. (A wet T-shirt offers even less protection.) A handful of innovative manufacturers are offering light-weight clothes that are specifically designed to offer additional sun protection. These garments are made of a tighter weave than is normally used, which blocks out most UV light. As of this writing, there are three manufacturers who claim that their outerwear offers an SPF of 30. In fact, one company has already received FDA approval to market their clothing line as official sun protection. (For a list of manufacturers, see Resources.)

ARTIFICIAL LIGHT

The sun is not the only source of UV light; artificial sources, such as florescent light, and halogen lamps can be equally dangerous. A plastic protective shield over a florescent bulb can prevent UV exposure. Older halogen lamps are more dangerous than the newer ones, which now come with plastic acrylic diffusers that absorb UV light. Halogen desk lamps in which the light is reflected down are the most dangerous in terms of UV exposure.

SELF-TANNING PRODUCTS

Some women may not want to be pale during the summer, and for them, self-tanning creams may be perfectly safe. The active ingredient in these creams is dihydroxyacetone, a dye that is absorbed into the skin and undergoes a chemical conversion that makes pigment.

Self-tanning creams were introduced several years ago, and the color was often on the sickly, orange side. Today, new tanning creams offer a more natural look. If you do opt for a self-tanning cream, keep in mind that it needs to be applied with great care or the result will be a streaky, uneven look. In fact, some beauty salons will apply it for you for a fee. (In New York, it costs about seventy dollars per application.)

Remember that although you look tan, you're really not tan, and are not any more protected from the sun than if you were pale. You must still wear your sun protection at all times. (If you have particularly sensitive skin, check with your doctor before using a self-tanning product.)

EYE CARE

Lupus as well as some of the medications used to control lupus can cause many different eye problems. For example, many lupus patients have Sjogren's syndrome, characterized by dry eyes. Hydroxychloroquine (Plaquenil) can affect the retina, and steroids can promote cataracts. It is essential for lupus patients to be aware of these potential problems and to take particular care of their eyes.

If you have mild disease and are not taking any medication, a careful eye examination by your own primary care physician should be done annually. However, if you are taking Plaquenil or steroids or have dry eye or other eye problems, you should be checked at least every six months by an ophthalmologist.

If you notice any of the following symptoms, call your doctor immediately.

    ✍ RED EYE. A sore, red eye could be a sign of any number of problems, including conjunctivitis (eye infection); episcleritis, an inflammation of the outer layers of the sclera, the white of the eye; or iritis, inflammation of an inner chamber of the eye that can occur in lupus patients. Don't self-medicate with over-the-counter eye drops. Go to your doctor for a thorough examination.

🙚 CHANGE IN VISION. If you notice that your vision is blurry or you see flashing lights or streaks or your vision is failing, call your doctor.

🙚 LIGHT SENSITIVITY. If you suddenly develop photophobia, a sensitivity to light, check with your doctor.

🙚 DRY, GRITTY EYES. If your eyes are becoming dry and gritty, call your doctor. It could be a sign of Sjogren's syndrome, or it could be caused by any number of medications. If you already have Sjogren's syndrome or chronically dry eyes, you are at an increased risk for corneal abrasion, a painful condition caused by the scratching of the cornea by soot or other particles that tears would normally wash away.

SUNGLASSES

If you have dry eyes, sunglasses are also very important because they protect against dust and other particles that can injure the vulnerable cornea. Heat and wind can also be very irritating, so wear the glasses even on days when it is not particularly sunny. Wraparound glasses with side shields offer additional protection, and some of them are quite stylish looking.

Women on steroids should also wear sunglasses; the combination of steroids and UV light can promote cataracts. Blocking UVA light may also diminish the risk of eye damage from antimalarial drugs. Not all sunglasses protect against UVA and UVB. Be sure to buy sunglasses that specifically promise to block 99 to 100 percent of UVA and UVB. If the label is confusing, check with your ophthalmologist. Be sure that the glasses fit well; UV rays can sneak in through gaps in glasses that are too loose or too small. Wear a hat in the sun; a hat with a wide brim can block about 50 percent of UV light.

CONTACT LENSES

Many women with lupus should avoid using contact lenses. In the case of Sjogren's syndrome, there is too great a risk of corneal abrasion or infection. (Soft lenses are no better than hard lenses. In fact, they actually absorb even more moisture from the eyes than hard lenses.) Even if you don't have dry eyes, lupus patients need to be careful about using contacts, especially those who are on immunosuppressive drugs that can reduce their resistance to infection. If you and your doctor agree that you can use contacts, be sure to be scrupulous about keeping your lenses clean. Disposable lenses may be best in some cases.

CLIMATE CONTROL

People with dry eyes should avoid overheated or overair-conditioned rooms that can further dry out their eyes. In some cases, a humidifier may help to add moisture to the air. Patients should avoid sitting under a hot hair dryer or drying their hair with a blow dryer for prolonged periods of time. Environments that are naturally dry, such as airplane cabins or areas that are in high altitudes, may be very irritating for people with dry eyes.

In any climate or altitude, dry eyes can be very uncomfortable, but there are a wide range of products available that can help to replace moisture; talk to your physician about which ones are right for you.

DENTAL CARE

Although everyone should practice good dental hygiene, it is especially important for women with lupus to be diligent about caring for their teeth and gums. It's critical to see your dentist at least every six months for a routine cleaning and examination. If you feel any pain in your mouth or notice any ulcers or abscesses, call your dentist or doctor immediately. If you are on immunosuppressive drugs, be extra careful about preventing gum infections, which in your immunosuppressed state will take longer to heal than normal and could spread to other areas.

DRY MOUTH

Many women with lupus have Sjogren's syndrome, or dry mouth, which can leave them prone to dental caries and gum disease. Certain medications can also cause dry mouth. Saliva not only moisturizes teeth, but has natural bacteria-fighting properties. People who do not have enough saliva run a greater risk of getting cavities and gum infections. Therefore, patients with dry mouth need to take meticulous care of their teeth. Brushing after every meal and daily flossing are essential. (If you can't brush, at least rinse your mouth out with water.) I recommend that patients use a fluoride rinse, such as Fluoroguard, daily to strengthen teeth. An antiplaque rinse, such as Plax, may help eliminate plaque formation, which can promote decay and gum disease. Try to avoid sweets, but if you can't, be sure to brush after eating a sugary treat.

Drinking frequent sips of water will help moisturize your mouth. Avoid sugary liquids, such as juice, soda, or sweetened coffee or tea; they'll only promote tooth decay. If you're mouth is very dry, your physician or dentist may prescribe oral pilocarpine, a pill that helps to promote saliva formation. Synthetic saliva sprays are also helpful (see p. 61). Chewing sugarless gum or sucking on sugarless candies or slippery elm bark cough drops may also help moisturize your mouth.

YEAST INFECTIONS

If your mouth or throat is very sore, it is possible that you have developed a yeast infection in the mouth (thrush), which is common with dry mouth or immunosuppression. Your doctor may prescribe an antifungal medication, such as Nystatin rinse or Mycelex troches.

CHAPTER 6

Maintaining a Healthy Lifestyle

Although being vigilant about monitoring yourself for signs of trouble and going for periodic checkups are essential for good health, these are not enough. Maintaining a healthy lifestyle is equally important for both your physical and emotional well-being. The following sections provide guidelines for living well with lupus.

GET ENOUGH SLEEP

Getting enough sleep is not a luxury, it is an absolute necessity for anyone with lupus. Recent studies show that sleep is intricately connected with the immune system, and in fact, sleep deprivation may cause the immune system to malfunction. Although the exact mechanism is still not understood, we do know that people who are sleep deprived are more prone to get sick. We also know that sleep has an anti-inflammatory effect on the body, although we don't know why.

If you have SLE, it is important for you to arrange your schedule to ensure that you get an adequate amount of sleep. Some women may be able to get by on eight hours, others may require more. Although an occasional late night may not hurt you, it's advisable not to make a practice of it. Nor is it advisable to push yourself to the point of exhaustion. When you are tired and want to go to sleep, your body is sending you a powerful message, and you should not ignore it.

LEARN TO CONTROL STRESS

Although there is no scientific evidence directly linking stress as a risk factor for SLE, there is a lot of anecdotal evidence suggesting that stress may indeed play a role in this disease. Rheumatologists have long observed that patients often have flares after experiencing a trauma or emotional turmoil in their lives, and studies show that stress can adversely affect the immune system.

Although no one is free from stress, there are ways to learn how to better cope with it. If you're experiencing a particularly difficult time, counseling from a mental health professional can help you learn how to deal with your problems in a constructive way. Exercise is also a wonderful way to relieve stress, and so is pursuing hobbies or outside activities that provide some enjoyment in your life.

If you feel stressed out, don't try to grin and bear it. Talk to your doctor for suggestions about where you can go for help, or call your local chapters of the Lupus Foundation or the Arthritis Foundation.

DON'T SMOKE

Although the rate of smoking is declining nationwide, it is actually rising among young women—and young women are the ones who are most likely to get lupus. Although smoking is very dangerous for all women, it is one vice that women with lupus should absolutely shun. First, smoking increases the odds of developing blood clots, which could result in stroke or heart attack. Women with antiphospholipid antibodies are already at a much higher risk of developing blood clots—smoking is merely adding fuel to the fire. Second, all women with lupus are also at greater risk of developing heart disease later in life. Smoking can promote atherosclerosis, high blood pressure, and heart attack. Smoking also damages your respiratory system (so can lupus) and can contribute to osteoporosis, another condition that women with lupus are more prone to develop. Smoking also increases your risk of developing peptic ulcer disease; patients on NSAIDs are already at increased risk for this problem. In addition, the nicotine in tobacco can cause spasms of arteries that can severely worsen Raynaud's symptoms. For this reason, the nicotine patch may be inadvisable for some lupus patients.

All in all, smoking is just plain dangerous and should be avoided. If you do smoke, call your local chapter of the Lung Association to find a smoking cessation program (see Resources or check in your local yellow pages).

AVOID EXCESSIVE ALCOHOL INTAKE

As long as your doctor says it's okay, an occasional alcoholic beverage is probably not harmful. However, keep in mind that many women with arthritic symptoms complain that alcohol actually makes their symptoms worse. In addition, women on NSAIDs may find alcohol very irritating to their stomachs, increasing the risk of gastritis and ulcers. Too much alcohol can also contribute to high cholesterol levels, a problem that many women with lupus are prone to develop. Although there have been studies that show that moderate drinking (one glass of wine daily for women) may help raise high-density lipoproteins, or "good cholesterol," in women, more than that may actually raise blood lipids to unhealthy levels. Three or four drinks a day can cause an unhealthy rise in blood pressure, which can contribute to heart and renal disease. Excessive drinking—certainly more than two drinks daily—may interfere with calcium and vitamin D absorption, which could contribute to osteoporosis.

There is also a danger that women who are under a great deal of stress, feeling lonely, or in pain may turn to alcohol (or other drugs) to help them cope. Women, especially older women, are often hidden drinkers. They indulge in the privacy of their homes and can go on for years before their problem is detected by family members or their physicians. Alcohol dependency is a serious problem for any woman, but it can certainly complicate a condition such as lupus. Women who suspect that they may have a problem with alcohol should seek help immediately. Talk to your doctor, or call a self-help group such as Alcoholics Anonymous (see Resources or check in your local yellow pages).

AVOID RECREATIONAL DRUGS

When you have a disease such as lupus, you shouldn't take any unnecessary risks with your body, and using recreational drugs can be very risky. Cocaine is particularly dangerous for women. Women's arteries are more prone to spasm than are men's—a problem that can be aggravated by cocaine—which can increase the risk of having a heart attack or stroke. In addition, women with Raynaud's already have arterial problems; the combination of Raynaud's and cocaine can be devastating.

Other recreational drugs may cause equally dangerous side effects and may be laced with impurities that may aggravate your symptoms or may be harmful, especially in combination with other medication.

MAINTAIN GOOD NUTRITION

In general, women with lupus should follow the advice offered by groups such as the American Heart Association and the American Cancer Society, who recommend that all Americans eat a "prudent diet."

- A prudent diet is basically a low-fat diet in which no more than 25 to 30 percent of calories come from fat.
- Limit salt intake to under 2,500 milligrams daily. (Reducing salt is especially important for women who retain fluid or have high blood pressure.)
- Eat fiber-rich foods—complex carbohydrates such as grains, legumes, fruits, and vegetables.
- Go lean on meat. Small portions of fish, poultry, and low-fat cuts of meat are permissible.
- Women with kidney disease should be especially careful about limiting their protein intake (meat, dairy products), which can stress the kidneys.

It is extremely important for lupus patients to be vigilant about controlling their fat intake for several reasons. First, fat is loaded with calories. One gram of fat weighs in at 9 calories; protein and carbohydrate are only 4 calories per gram. Obviously, you can eat a lot more nonfat food for a lot less calories. Weight control is a common problem for women with lupus, especially for those on steroids, which are appetite-enhancing. Steroids actually stimulate the gastric juices in the stomach, which make you feel hungry. If you crave food, look for snacks low in calories and fat. Quelling hunger with a piece of fruit like a banana, a rice cake with jam, or vegetables dipped into a low-fat yogurt dressing will not put on weight; eating high-fat, sugary snack foods will most definitely add on the pounds. In addition, complex carbohydrates take longer to digest and leave you feeling fuller longer than high-fat, sugary foods that are quickly broken down.

Second, many lupus patients, particularly those on steroids or with kidney abnormalities, are at greater risk of developing high cholesterol levels. Certain forms of fat, notably saturated fat, which is found primarily in meat and dairy products, can raise cholesterol levels in the body. Studies show that for women, cholesterol levels over 230 milligrams per deciliter significantly increase the risk of having a heart attack. Therefore, it is important to try to keep cholesterol levels under 230.

Maintaining a high intake of calcium and vitamin D is essential to help prevent osteoporosis: Vitamin D promotes calcium absorption. Women who have been on steroids are at greater risk of developing this degenerative disease, but it is a problem that all women need to be concerned about. Several studies have shown that few women get the 1,200 milligrams of calcium they need daily to maintain healthy bones (1,500 milligrams after menopause). Up until around age thirty, women create new bone tissue each year, resulting in their peak bone mass. After age forty, women begin to lose some of their bone mass each year. Calcium in combination with vitamin D may help stem some of this bone loss.

Getting an adequate amount of calcium and vitamin D can be difficult. Women with lupus are advised to avoid the sun and, therefore, miss a major source of natural vitamin D. (The rays of sun that stimulate the formation of vitamin D in the body are filtered out by sunscreens.) It's imperative for women to drink vita-

∽ GOOD FOR YOUR BONES. Weight-bearing exercise, the kind of exercise that works muscles and bones against gravity, helps to maintain bone mass, which can prevent osteoporosis or thinning of the bones. After age thirty-five, women lose bone mass at a rate of 1 percent each year; after menopause, they lose about 5 percent of bone mass per year. The rate of bone loss may be even more in women who are or have been on steroids. Several studies have shown that women who exercise maintain significantly more bone mass than women who are sedentary.

∽ WEIGHT CONTROL. Exercise burns calories, which helps to maintain normal weight.

∽ GOOD FOR YOUR EMOTIONAL WELL-BEING. Exercise helps to release stress, which is good for your cardiovascular and mental health. There is also some anecdotal evidence that stress may aggravate lupus, although as of yet, there is no scientific proof. In addition, vigorous exercise (fast walking, running) helps release endorphins, chemicals in the brain that help control pain and foster a feeling of well-being.

∽ BUILDS STAMINA. When you exert yourself during exercise, your heart beats faster and has to work harder. As a result, it becomes stronger and better able to handle the demands that are placed on it daily.

∽ BUILDS BODY CONFIDENCE. Exercise helps you to feel good about your body even though it may not be "perfect." It is especially important for women with lupus not to dwell on their physical limitations, but to develop good positive feelings about their physical selves.

Although exercise offers many benefits, it can be dangerous in certain situations. For example, high-impact aerobics is overly stressful to the knees and should be avoided especially in women who have arthritis or are on steroids.

Every woman should be able to do some kind of exercise. However, the level and type of exercise will depend on several factors. After being diagnosed with lupus, every woman should consider having at least one meeting with a physical therapist who can help her tailor an exercise program to meet her specific needs. For example, if you are severely ill or experiencing a flare, you should not overexert yourself. In these situations, rest can be very therapeutic. However, you can still do a regimen of mild range-of-motion exercises that allow you to gently extend and flex your joints as long as it is not too painful.

If you have mild disease, you can engage in a fairly normal exercise regimen. Ideally, you should do a combination of toning and stretching exercises for flexibility as well as walking or some other kind of weight-bearing exercise (running, tennis), which will help prevent osteoporosis. If you have knee, hip, or ankle arthritis, I would avoid running, jogging, using a stairmaster, or doing anything else that puts excessive pressure on your legs. Swimming is a wonderful exercise because it provides a cardiovascular workout and allows for full range of motion for most joints in a weightless environment. Many patients who find other exercise painful are able to enjoy swimming. However, because it is not a weight-bearing exercise, it does not help to maintain bone mass.

Some lupus patients have found that yoga offers them excellent toning and stretching as well as promoting deep relaxation.

If you can manage it, walking at a brisk rate for a mile or two daily is excellent because it strengthens muscles and bones and provides a good cardiovascular workout. It is also relatively safe and enjoyable. (If you've never exercised before or are over forty, check with your doctor before starting any exercise program.) If you're beginning a walking program, begin slowly by walking a few blocks daily, gradually building up your endurance to a full mile each way. If possible, walk with a companion—it's safer and more fun. Stop if you feel any pain, dizziness, shortness of breath, or heart palpitations and call your doctor. Be sure to wear sunscreen and a hat, even in cloudy weather. Many people who live in suburbs find large malls a good place to do their walking workout—no worry about sun there!

If you prefer to work out in a gym, avoid using any weights over 2 pounds—anything heavier is too stressful for your joints. In addition, keep in mind that your hands, which may have loose ligaments due to lupus, are particularly vulnerable to injury. Therefore, avoid exercises that put your weight on your fingertips, such as fingertip push-ups.

LOOKING GOOD

For many women, how they feel is inextricably linked to how well they look. Women with lupus are no different. Lupus, especially during active disease, can cause many physical changes that can make a woman feel quite unattractive. A prominent malar rash or hair loss due to lupus can be very disturbing. Weight gain, swelling, and the growth of facial hair from steroids can be extremely upsetting. In some cases, the changes in physical appearance can be quite profound. As one patient put it, "I know that it may sound vain, but sometimes the thing that gets to me the most is how lupus has changed my looks. It's hard not be upset by the fact that when I look in the mirror, I don't recognize my own face."

Fortunately, many of these physical changes are reversed when the flare subsides and/or when the medication dose can be reduced or even eliminated. However, that is small comfort to the woman who is in the midst of a flare or who needs to be maintained on high doses of medication and whose body image is being battered by her disease. Unfortunately, the impact of lupus on physical appearance has been somewhat ignored by the medical profession. Women with SLE often say that their doctors dismiss their negative feelings about their looks, especially if their problems are caused by medication, by reminding them that they are lucky to be living in a time when we can treat lupus so successfully. Although this may be true, it does little to repair the patient's damaged self-esteem. It's very important to encourage patients to try to look their best despite their illness. Looking good not only boosts a patient's morale and improves her outlook on life, but also helps her to channel some of her frustration and anger into a positive endeavor.

It's not easy to counter the cosmetic damage inflicted by lupus, and it can be time-consuming. However, women who devote the time and energy to looking good will look and feel a lot better. The following is some specific advice on how to tackle the most common problems caused by lupus.

ഛ MALAR RASH, STRETCH MARKS. There are several cosmetics on the market that are specifically designed to cover rashes and conspicuous blemishes. The Covermark line of cosmetics provides excellent coverage for hard-to-conceal rashes and blemishes. Many Covermark products also provide sun protection (SPF 16 to 20). Covermark also has leg makeup that can camouflage stretch marks (striae) in areas of sudden weight gain, which can be caused by steroids. Unlike normal stretch marks, these are a more noticeable lavender and reddish color. Dermablend is another cosmetic line that is designed to conceal the more conspicuous facial rashes and blemishes.

Both Covermark and Dermablend are sold in many department stores. Although these products work well, they do require a certain amount of skill to use them correctly. Finding the right skin shade and applying the makeup so that it is both effective and natural looking can be a bit challenging. Some department stores may have a trained cosmetologist working at the cosmetics counter who can demonstrate how to use these products correctly. Very often, if you purchase some makeup, the consultation is free. In addition, Covermark will provide counseling by phone (see Resources) and also has a videotape that provides tips on how to apply their makeup.

ᥱᥲ HAIR LOSS. Many women with lupus experience hair loss (alopecia) either from lupus or as a side effect from medication. In most cases, the hair will eventually grow back (the one exception is discoid lupus, which may cause permanent scarring that prevents regrowth). However, there is no reason to walk around feeling self-conscious or uncomfortable if you are losing your hair. There are now salons that specialize in styles for women with hair loss. Your dermatologist may be able to help steer you to them. The National Alopecia Areata Foundation (see Resources) provides excellent information on how to select a wig that is right for you. Call or write them for this information before purchasing a wig. It's important to note that the Alopecia Foundation stresses that an inexpensive synthetic wig ($59 to $125) can often work just as well as one that costs hundreds or even thousands of dollars more. In fact, synthetic wigs are actually easier to care for than those made of real human hair, which tend to be more expensive. Check with your insurance carrier to see if the cost of a wig may be covered as a prosthesis. Fashionable hats, turbans, and scarves offer attractive alternatives and may be more comfortable than a wig.

ఴ EXCESSIVE FACIAL HAIR. Steroids can cause excessive hair growth on the face. Fortunately, the unwanted hair can be handled in any number of ways. If it is very fine, bleaching may make the hair less noticeable. There are several commercial bleaches for facial hair that are sold at most drug stores and pharmacies. However, if the hair is very thick, bleaching may actually make it more noticeable. In this case, you may want to consider using a depilatory (hair remover), which is sold over the counter at most drug stores. Although most depilatories work well, the hair will grow back, and the chemicals used can be irritating to sensitive skin. Another option is waxing. Warm wax is poured over the hairy area. When the wax dries, it is peeled off, taking the hair with it. Waxing can be done at a beauty salon or at home. It is not permanent—the hair will grow back within a few weeks, although sometimes thinner than it was before—and waxing can be irritating to people with sensitive skin. A final choice is electrolysis, a permanent hair removal system in which a tiny needle is inserted into the root of each hair. A small electric shock is delivered into the root, killing the hair follicle. Electrolysis can be painful and irritating to people with sensitive skin, but it is permanent. It can also be expensive. Talk to your doctor about which hair removal system would be best for you.

ఴ GOOD GROOMING. No matter how bad you may feel, putting on makeup and slipping into an attractive outfit is going to make you feel better. So will wearing jewelry, getting manicures, and wearing or doing anything else that makes you feel a bit pampered or special. Perfume or fancy, scented soaps, lotions, powders, or bubble bath are relatively inexpensive ways to pamper yourself. When you're sick, it's very easy to let yourself go or to think, "I look so bad, why should I even bother?" But that's precisely the time that doing little things for yourself can make a big difference in both morale and outlook.

ON THE ROAD

I have many patients who travel routinely for work or for pleasure. Unless you are in the midst of a flare, there is no reason why you can't take normal vacations or go on business trips. However, to be on the safe side, I advise my patients to avoid countries with poor sanitation, a suspect water supply, or inferior medical facilities. Although in most cases, women with lupus can travel with little difficulty, they need to know that if they should get sick, they can get adequate care.

In addition, there some other precautions that you must take to ensure that you stay happy and healthy on the road.

✎ PLAN FOR AN EMERGENCY. Before you leave, you and your doctor should discuss what procedure to follow if you should develop a flare or other illness on your trip. Get the name of a physician or major medical center in the area where you will be traveling. If you're traveling in the United States, the national chapters of the Lupus and Arthritis Foundations can provide local referrals (see Resources). If you are taking steroids or have taken steroids within the past year, you should talk to your doctor about bringing additional doses in case of a flare.

✎ DON'T RUN OUT OF MEDICINE. Bring a double supply of medicine with you on all trips. Pack one in your carry-on luggage or pocketbook and one in your suitcase, just in case you lose one of your bags. If you've been on an NSAID in the past, talk to your doctor about bringing a supply of anti-inflammatory medicine with you in case you need it. In addition, bring a copy of your prescriptions as well as a letter from your physician summarizing your medical history.

✎ MAKE SURE THAT YOU HAVE HAD PROPER IMMUNIZATION FOR THE AREA IN WHICH YOU ARE TRAVELING. Check with your physician to be certain that the recommended shots do not interfere with your treatment.

✎ PROPHYLACTIC ANTIBIOTICS. I advise my patients to take a full course of antibiotics with them on all major trips in case they get sick. This is especially important for patients who are on immunosuppressive drugs. We discuss in detail when and how these drugs should be taken, and I ask them to call me before beginning the antibiotic regimen to determine if they really need it and/or if they should be seen by a doctor.

✎ STOMACH PROTECTION. Don't forget to bring along some antacids—new food and different water may cause stomach upset. (You may already have some stomach upset from your medication, especially if you're on NSAIDs.) In addition, bring some Immodium in case you get a case of traveler's diarrhea.

⚜ ANTIHISTAMINE. Pack some antihistamine in case you get an allergic reaction. Certain brands of antihistamine may cause dry mouth and dry eye. If you have Sjogren's syndrome or have problems with dry mouth or eye, talk to your physician or call the Sjogren's Foundation to find out which antihistamine is best for you.

⚜ BRING SUN PROTECTION. Obviously, if you're traveling to a warm, sunny climate, you need to be very careful about sun exposure. Keep in mind, the further south you go toward the equator, the stronger the sun's rays. Don't forget that if you're traveling to the Southern Hemisphere, the seasons are reversed—it's summer there when it's winter here. However, no matter where you may travel, be sure to pack your sunscreen, especially if you are going to a remote area where it may be difficult to buy any or they may not have a brand that works well for you.

⚜ GET TRIP INSURANCE. One of the most aggravating aspects of lupus is its unpredictability—it can strike at the most inconvenient times, like right before a trip. In many cases, you have to prepay for trips and getting your money back can be tricky, even if it's a legitimate excuse. Therefore, it's a good idea to purchase trip insurance, which is usually sold by travel agents or tour operators. Read the small print: Some policies exclude pre-existing conditions. Make sure the policy also covers your fare home and reimburses you for any money you might have prepaid (for hotels, tours, etc.) if you have to cut your trip short due to illness.

⚜ SPECIAL NEEDS. If you are disabled or require special attention or equipment (wheel chair, walker, etc.), alert the airline, tour operator, and so on before you embark on your journey. For more information, you should contact one of the many advocacy groups for the disabled that offer advice and information for disabled travelers (see Resources).

⚜ DON'T GET OVERTIRED. Traveling can throw you off your normal schedule. Be sure to allow for enough time to rest. If you require a nap in the afternoon or early evening at home, you should also plan for one while you're on the road. Don't try to cover too much territory at one time; the stress of changing cities and hotel rooms every few days may be too much for some people. Before embarking on a trip, give yourself plenty of time to pack and prepare, even if it means leaving a day or two later. For example, if you work full-time, you may not be able to race home after work and catch the midnight flight on Friday night, return the following week on Sunday, and be back at your job feeling well enough to work on Monday. A more sensible approach would be to plan to travel from Saturday to Saturday; this will enable you to travel to and from your destination at a more relaxed pace and will give you a day to rest before returning to work.

CHAPTER 7

Love and Lupus

Lupus is part of what I am. If he loves me, he has to accept my lupus.

—Mary, thirty-one, married for five years

Meeting the right man—one who is understanding, considerate, mature, and willing to commit—and sustaining a long-term relationship can be a challenge for any woman these days whether or not she has lupus. In this respect, women with lupus share many of the same problems as other women in the relationship arena; however, there are some important differences.

These differences can surface early in a relationship. When most women are preoccupied with questions like, Does he really like me? Do I like him? and Do we have enough in common? the woman with lupus is grappling with a far more difficult question: When do I tell him that I have lupus? During the initial stages of dating, you don't have to reveal too many details of your personal life, including your health status. It's not that you should be embarrassed or ashamed about having lupus, it's simply not a relevant topic of conversation in casual interaction. You don't expect a man to say, "I have a family history of heart disease, my cholesterol is too high, both my parents are bald, and I'm at risk of having a heart attack before I'm fifty" on the first date. In fact, if he did, you would probably be put off, not so much by the confession, but by the fact that he didn't have anything more interesting to talk about. You and your date hopefully have full enough lives and enough in common that you could spend an evening or two together without having to talk about illness—either yours or his.

GETTING SERIOUS

If you begin to get serious with someone, it's time to have a frank discussion about lupus. At the very least, someone who you spend a lot of time with needs to understand your physical restrictions (if there are any) and what activities may contribute to a flare. For instance, if you need a full eight hours of sleep a night not to feel too fatigued the next day, your date should respect that and not push you to overextend yourself. Or if you need to stay out of the sun, your date should not insist on spending every waking minute of the summer at the beach. In most cases, it is not unreasonable to ask a friend to accommodate your needs—even women without lupus may have certain restrictions on their time or activities. Some women may have to work weekends, others may be fair skinned and need to avoid the sun, still others may be highly allergic and prefer to spend hay fever season in an air-conditioned room. You shouldn't feel as if you're imposing on your friendship by asking someone to consider your well-being.

If someone is unwilling to accommodate you in any way, it is a good sign that he is simply not mature enough to handle the situation. Not everyone will be. In fact, if your goal is to get married, you will have to go out of your way to look for a serious and down-to-earth person. A man in his early twenties who is still unsettled may not be a good choice unless he is very mature for his age. Someone who is a bit older and has had more life experience may be better able to understand that life is full of twists and turns and that even if you marry someone with a clean bill of health, it doesn't mean that you are "safe" from adversity.

When you tell your boyfriend about lupus, don't expect that he will understand what you are saying, at least initially. For one thing, he may not want to hear it. He may view you in a very romantic way—as a girlfriend, a lover, and possibly as a potential wife. The last thing that he wants to hear about is an illness getting in the way of his dreams. For another, it may seem very unreal, particularly if you look well and don't have any obvious symptoms.

Most young people in their teens and twenties have had very little experience with illness. In many cases, their parents are still relatively healthy, and they may even have two sets of living grandparents. Unless your boyfriend has had personal experience with illness, he will probably not fully comprehend the potential impact of a chronic disease on your life and future relationship. In fact, very likely, your boyfriend will not accept what you are telling him and may enter a phase of denial, similar to the one that you experienced when you first learned that you had lupus. He may prefer to proceed as if he didn't know that you had a chronic illness, and it may be tempting for you both to sweep the truth under the rug. However, if you are planning to marry, for the sake of the future relationship, you must both fully understand what you are getting into. Before you make serious plans for the future, here are some issues that must be addressed:

☙ FULL DISCLOSURE. Your future husband should have a clear and full understanding of the medical aspects of lupus in general and your case in particular. Encourage him to read this book. Make an appointment for you and him to sit down with your doctor and have a straightforward, honest conversation. If you have mild disease and your doctor believes that it will probably stay that way, your future partner still needs to be aware of possible complications down the road, for instance, the possibility that you may have a flare during pregnancy. If you have a more serious case, for example, if you have a history of kidney disease and frequent hospitalizations, your future husband must fully understand the implications of your diagnosis and the possibility that you could get a lot sicker.

☙ CHILDREN. Although many women with lupus can have children with little or no problem, there is always the possibility that you may not be as lucky. Your future husband needs to be know that pregnancy may possibly aggravate your condition, or if you are not well enough, your doctor may advise against it. He also needs to know that he must be prepared to be a hands-on father; if you flare during or after pregnancy, you may need extra help until you are back on your feet.

ௐ FINANCES. Many families today rely on two paychecks to make ends meet. Even though you may be feeling fine now and able to work, there may be times when you may have to work part-time or not at all. Your future husband needs to acknowledge that he may have to be the primary breadwinner, at least some of the time, and you need to adjust your lifestyle accordingly.

ௐ COUNSELING—ALONE AND TOGETHER. You and your fiancé should get some couples' counseling before you get married, preferably from a marriage counselor, psychologist, or social worker who is familiar with chronic illness. The counseling will not only provide an outlet to voice your concerns about the future, but will help develop the communications skills that you will need to sustain your marriage, especially through difficult times.

Your fiancé may have a lot of questions and fears that he may not want to voice in front of you. He may be worried about having to care for you if you get sick and whether or not he could handle the pressure. He may be worried that you won't be able to have a normal sex life or he may be fearful that his children will be born sick (in most cases, they'll be fine). Encourage him to talk with other knowledgeable people who can answer his questions and quiet his fears. Call the Lupus Foundation and see if they can put him in contact with a supportive (and happily married) husband who can talk about living with a woman with lupus. He may also need to seek some counseling on his own; if he does, don't feel betrayed by his fears. It is far better for both of you that he work through his reservations before you are married than to have them surface sometime down the road.

DEALING WITH PARENTS AND IN-LAWS

When you're planning to get married, the last thing you want to hear is anyone expressing doubts about your decision, especially your fiancé's parents. However, once your future in-laws learn that you have a chronic illness, they may be very worried about what the future has in store for their son, and they may openly express their fears. Both you and your fiancé may feel hurt and angered by their doubts, and this may cause a serious rift in your relationship with his parents. Despite your initial feelings, I urge you to be patient and understanding with them. Don't take their reservations about your marriage personally—it's only natural for parents to be protective toward their child. Your fiancé's parents may be very scared that their son is getting into something that he may not be able to handle.

Your job is to educate your future in-laws. Make sure that they understand that most women with lupus lead fairly normal lives and that even if you get sick, in all likelihood your symptoms can be controlled through medication. If your in-laws are uncomfortable asking you about lupus, perhaps you can get them together with your parents, who may be able to answer some of their questions. Perhaps you can also refer them to the Lupus Foundation for information and counseling.

In the best of circumstances, some parents may be upset at the prospect of losing a child to marriage. It may take time for them to adjust to the idea of their son as an independent adult with his own family. Try not to become alienated from them during this difficult time—you may need their support down the road.

Depending on your situation, your parents may also be less than thrilled by your decision to marry. They may say things like, "What if you get sick? Do you think he'll take care of you?" or "You're doing so well now, why would you want to get pregnant and take that risk?" Their doubts about your ability to be a wife and mother may hurt you very deeply and may erode your confidence in yourself and your future husband. You may strike back by becoming angry and defensive.

Understanding why your parents feel the way they do may help put their objections in perspective. Very often, parents become overprotective of their children, viewing them as fragile and vulnerable well into adulthood. These are the same parents who may have had to nurse you through many illnesses and who fretted over your every symptom. They are terrified that you are going to get sick, and they will not be able to do anything about it. They are deeply concerned that your future husband will not have the backbone to stick it out if things get rough and that, in the end, you will be hurt. Deep down they believe that no one will take care of you as well as they did. (In that respect, they're right, but adults don't need to be cared for like children.) They have latched on to all of these fears in addition to the normal ones that parents typically feel when a daughter strikes out on her own.

Even if the daughter goes ahead and marries, she may still be overly dependent on her parents, which may intrude on her relationship with her husband. In this situation, professional counseling can be invaluable in helping the daughter and her parents learn how to relate to each other as adults and in helping her parents accept her marriage.

There are times, however, when your parents or future in-laws may sense that your fiancé may not be up to the task of living with someone with a chronic illness. Your parents may point out that your fiancé has been inconsiderate or unavailable every time you've been sick. Your future mother-in-law may tell you that her son falls apart in hospitals and can't stand being around illness. Although these kinds of things may be painful to hear, you need to listen and honestly ask yourself whether there is any truth to them. If you can't unequivocally say, "Oh, he's always been there for me" or "He's not like that," be sure to bring up these issues during premarital counseling. You don't have to call off the wedding if he is less than perfect; however, you need to be aware of your fiancé's weaknesses as well as his strengths.

PRESSURES ON AN EXISTING MARRIAGE

In a way, it may be easier for the couple if the wife has been diagnosed before they marry and they have some familiarity with lupus. In this case, both partners have some sense of what lies ahead and have embarked upon the journey together willingly. It can be far more difficult for the relationship if the woman gets sick during an existing marriage, which can radically change both roles and expectations for both husband and wife. A man who is used to being cared for by his wife in many ways may now be placed in the role of caregiver, a role in which he may not feel comfortable. Suddenly, in addition to being breadwinner, the husband of a wife who has become ill may also be forced to assume the responsibility of running the household and caring for the children. If in addition to maintaining the household, the wife also worked outside the home, the family may be missing the second paycheck if she is too ill to return to work. These changes can put an enormous stress on a marriage.

It can also be extremely tough for the husband of a newly diagnosed woman to fully comprehend the chronic nature of lupus. Typically, when a wife gets sick enough to take to her bed, such as in the case of the flu, most husbands are willing to pitch in during the time when she is acutely ill. They'll change diapers, cook dinner, and wash dishes until their wife gets better. Then, when she's back on her feet, the couple will usually revert back to their old habits and roles. However, lupus is fairly unpredictable, and many women fluctuate dramatically from day to day. One day they'll feel well, the next day they'll be too tired to get out of bed. It's certainly not pleasant for the patient, but it can be very discouraging for the spouse who may feel that life will never get back to normal or at least the way it was before his wife got sick. As one woman who was diagnosed with lupus two years ago notes, "Before I got sick, I did everything. I did the yard work, I ran the household, and I also worked. I had a lot of energy back then. When I was first diagnosed, my husband did help out a lot. But now he doesn't. I'm not sick every day, but there are days that I just can't even put the laundry in the machine or clear the dishes out of the sink. He waits for me to do it no matter what. When I try to talk about lupus, he won't listen. My husband just can't accept the fact that I'm sick or that this is something that may last forever."

This husband is obviously in an intense stage of denial, which is seriously threatening his marriage. His wife is very bitter about his reaction and feels emotionally abandoned. Her husband is desperately trying to hold onto the past and to resume a "normal life." It is difficult for him to accept that their lives together have changed. Like the couple who is contemplating marriage, this couple needs counseling by a person who is experienced with chronic illness. Despite his fears and objections, the husband needs to become educated about lupus, and his wife needs to better understand his feelings.

Even if a couple enters into marriage after diagnosis, they may run into problems when theory becomes reality. Some of these marriages will not survive the pressure of a chronic illness, but some may not have survived anyway. Divorce is not unusual in our society. Although the divorce rate is somewhat higher among people with chronic illnesses, any stress, from infertility to unemployment, is going to take its toll on a marriage. It requires a great deal of understanding and hard work on the part of both partners to hold a marriage together, particularly one that is under stress, but a determined couple can do it. I know many who have and whose marriages would be considered successful whether or not they had lupus.

In preparation for this chapter, I have talked with several happily married women with lupus and asked them why they feel that their marriages have withstood the strain of chronic illness. Based on their interviews and my experiences with my patients, I have come up with the following advice.

❧ DON'T LET THE MARRIAGE REVOLVE AROUND ILLNESS. When one partner in a marriage is sick, it is very easy for the marriage—and the household—to become fixated on the illness. There are times when a couple may find their only excursions together are to the doctor's office and their only topic of conversation is lupus. This is not good for you or your husband. It is critical that you both maintain other interests. You need to keep up your friendships, even if at times it's only by telephone. Encourage your husband to try to keep up with his friends and his hobbies.

Try to find at least one special activity that you can do together on a regular basis. Because your husband may have to accommodate your needs very often, this is a good opportunity for you to reciprocate. Pick something that he is enthusiastic about. For example, if he loves basketball or tennis, go to some games with him. If he's a movie buff, get a subscription for a foreign film festival. If you're both interested in the arts, sign up for a related course at a local college or art center. Unless you are acutely sick, you should be able to pursue some activity that will allow you both to focus on something other than lupus.

❧ MAINTAIN YOUR COUPLENESS. During times of acute illness, intimacy seems to disappear. Members of your extended family or friends may be hovering around your home, caring for you or helping out with the kids. During this period, it is very important for a couple to maintain their "coupleness." You may not be able to go out to dinner or to a movie, but you can certainly shut your bedroom door, turn off the phone, and spend some quality time together. Send the children off to someone's house for a few hours or get a sitter. For a treat, order out from your favorite restaurant or bring in some videos. Whatever you do, don't let anyone intrude on your private time together.

⮞ HE NEEDS SUPPORT, TOO. You may be the one who is sick, but your husband's life has also been profoundly affected by lupus. At times, he's going to be as angry and frustrated as you are, and he will need support. As one woman who has been happily married for eight years so eloquently explains, "When we talk to people about lupus, it's almost as if it's happening to both of us, not just me. You don't know how many times my husband has said to me, 'I know that it's you who are going through everything and who's feeling everything physically, but I'm going through as much as you're going through.' I know that there are times when he thinks about the way things used to be, and he gets very angry that this had to happen. There are times that he'll say to other people, 'I sometimes feel like I just want to crawl into a hole and hide.' That's just how the sick person feels. It's only normal when the person that you love feels frustrated about what you're going through. When this happens, don't get on his case, let him talk about it. He needs to work it through."

⮞ DON'T EXPECT HIM TO READ YOUR MIND. A woman tends to think that if a man really loves her, he will somehow intuitively know how she feels and what she needs. Part of this stems from the fact that many women have a very difficult time asserting their needs. One of the hardest tasks for a woman is to simply state what she wants in clear, understandable language. When a woman has lupus and has many needs, this inability to express her needs can create some real problems in her marriage. One mother of two recalled, "I used to grit my teeth, try to do everything by myself, race around the house like a normal wife and mother to prove that I could be Superwoman, and then when I felt completely exhausted and overwhelmed, I would explode at my husband." This couple finally went to see a counselor who specialized in chronic illness and helped them devise a better way of communicating. "We've become very proactive, we just don't wait for things to happen. Instead of me screaming later, we work things out ahead of time. I don't wait for him to volunteer, instead I say, 'Let's talk about the weekend. How are we going to manage to take the kids to two soccer games and who's going to shop for the birthday presents?' And when I can't do something, I let him know. I used to have the responsibility of getting the kids dressed for school, making their breakfasts, and packing their lunches while I was trying to shower and get dressed to go to work. It was too much for me. Instead of me screaming, 'You bastard, you never help me,' I finally told my husband precisely what I needed him to do. Now he packs the lunches and makes breakfast for the kids. It has made a huge difference in my life and in our relationship."

Good communication is the most important factor in any marriage, but the stakes are even higher when you are in a high-stress situation. As difficult as it may be for you to say and at times for him to hear, most men would prefer a straightforward comment than having to constantly guess what you are thinking and feeling.

⤜ DON'T HAVE UNREALISTIC EXPECTATIONS. Patients often complain that during times when they are acutely ill, their husbands are very attentive to their needs—they'll cook dinner and drive the kids to school—but then, when they improve, their husbands quickly revert to their old ways. This often causes a lot of resentment on the part of women who wish their husbands would be that helpful all the time. As I said previously, if there's something that you specifically need from your husband, you should ask for it. However, I would keep in mind that you can't always expect him to be Superman. Most men don't do housework unless they are specifically asked—just ask your friends about what goes on in their homes. If your husband comes through when you really need him, don't be angry when he behaves like a "normal man" the rest of the time.

⤜ MAINTAIN YOUR SEXUAL RELATIONSHIP. Sexual dysfunction is not an uncommon problem in a chronic illness such as lupus. There are times when you may be in pain or feel too fatigued or depressed to feel sexy. Other related problems such as vaginal dryness or a yeast infection may interfere with sexual pleasure. All of this is understandable, and yet it is very important to your relationship that you try to maintain a regular sex life.

The physical problems are actually the easiest to overcome. Vaginal dryness can be helped by using a personal lubricant during intercourse; a yeast infection can usually be easily remedied by an antifungal medication, many of which are sold over the counter. If you're fatigued at night, you can have sex in the early evening or afternoon. If you have joint or hip pain you can take a warm bath before sex to ease the pain, and stick to positions that do not put pressure on painful joints. For more information, talk to your doctor or read *The Guide to Independent Living for People with Arthritis*, published by the Arthritis Foundation, which provides some excellent advice on sexuality (see Resources).

The emotional roadblocks to a fulfilling sex life may be more difficult to surmount. If your body has undergone changes from medication, such as steroids, or the lupus itself, you may feel unattractive and undesirable. Making an effort to look attractive despite your physical problems is the first step toward affirming your sexuality. Good communication between you and your partner is also essential. Very often, a lack of understanding between partners can interfere with normal sexuality. Enid Englehardt of the SLE Foundation in New York, a social worker who often counsels couples, recalls this telling story. Recently, she met with a distraught young woman who said that ever since she had a lupus flare on her honeymoon six months ago, her husband has not made any romantic overtures. When Ms. Englehardt met with the woman's husband, he confessed that he was afraid to have sex with his wife because he believed that it would be too painful for her. Fortunately, through counseling, the couple finally resolved their differences and resumed their sex life.

Maintaining your sex life is not only good for your emotional well-being, but it's also good for your physical health. Recent studies show that sexual activity may actually strengthen your immune system, decrease stress, and relieve arthritic symptoms. (Sexual activity may release chemicals called *endorphins*, nature's own natural pain relievers.) Another major study showed that couples with a fulfilling sex life were less hostile toward each other and less likely to blame each other for their problems.

❧ GIVE HIM SOME TIME OFF. When you have a disease such as lupus, there are certain restrictions in your life that you take for granted. If you are photosensitive, you avoid the sun; if you have joint pain or fatigue, there are times that you may avoid certain forms of intense physical exercise. Keep in mind, however, that you should not expect your spouse to curtail his activities in quite the same way. There are several ways that loving couples can work this out to their mutual benefit. Cindy, who has bad arthritis, makes it a point to go on vacation with another couple so her husband has people to do things with when she needs to rest. "I know that I'm limited in what I can do, and I want my husband to be able to do some of the things that he enjoys. This way, I don't feel guilty or that I'm letting him down if I want to go back to the room and take a nap," she explained.

Another woman, Laura, whose husband, John, has been very supportive of her through the years, has found a way to show him her appreciation. A great outdoor enthusiast, John believes that the word *vacation* is synonymous with white-water rafting and long, arduous hikes in the woods. Since Laura can no longer accompany him on these trips, she encourages him to take a camping vacation with his male friends every other year. As difficult as it is for her to care for their two children on her own while John is away, Laura says it is well worth the effort. "It's such an important thing to him. He comes back so refreshed and full of love and ready to be reciprocal, and he has the next trip to look forward to. He has such a good time planning for it with his friends that I think that it carries him through the bad times."

✑ GET HELP WHEN YOU NEED IT. When things get rough, don't assume that you can handle it on your own. Sometimes the everyday problems of family living can be difficult; add lupus into the picture, and they can be overwhelming. Very often, counseling from a trained professional who is experienced with chronic illness can get you and your spouse back on track.

CHAPTER 8

Pregnancy:
The Odds Are in Your Favor

Until the past decade or so, conventional wisdom dictated that women with SLE should not have children; in fact, if pregnancy did occur, many doctors recommended therapeutic abortion. Back then, doctors believed that pregnancy automatically triggered a flare, which would seriously imperil the health of both mother and baby. We now know that they were wrong. For the majority of women with SLE, motherhood is an achievable goal. Under the right conditions, most women with lupus can get through pregnancy with few, if any, problems and will deliver normal, healthy babies. However, in order to have a happy outcome, lupus mothers must plan carefully for pregnancy and must be closely monitored by their physicians from conception to delivery. Very little should be left to chance.

I strongly believe that women with SLE should be vigilant enough about their own health to prevent accidental pregnancy. Getting pregnant at the wrong time, for instance, during a flare, could result in a miscarriage or stillbirth as well as in serious complications for the mother.

The decision of whether or not to bear a child is a highly personal one. Some women are willing to take great risks to become mothers, others are not. Your doctor, family, and close friends can offer advice, but ultimately the choice is yours. If you are infertile or if you and your physician decide that pregnancy may be detrimental to your health, adoption may be a viable alternative.

In order to make an informed choice, there are several factors that must be considered by women before embarking on a pregnancy.

YOUR PREPREGNANCY CHECKLIST

Maternal health. Although pregnancy is a natural and normal phenomenon, it puts an enormous strain on a woman's body. In order to nourish the new life, every single organ system in your body must work 50 percent harder than normal. Therefore, it is important to start a pregnancy from a position of strength. The prospective mother should be in stable medical condition for at least six months before becoming pregnant, that is, in remission or with minimal disease. If possible, her renal function should be close to normal; kidneys are particularly vulnerable during pregnancy. If she has had a history of renal disease, her condition should be stabilized and well controlled.

It is crucial to time your pregnancy to coincide with periods of good health. A recent study showed that if lupus is inactive at the time of conception, there is a 70 percent chance that it will remain inactive. However, if a woman with active disease becomes pregnant, there is a 40 percent chance that it will get worse and an equal chance that it will stay the same. A small number will improve.

What drugs are you taking? Since many drugs can cross the placenta and cause birth defects, the potential mother should be taking as little medication as possible prior to conception. If you're taking medication and planning to become pregnant, talk to your physician about potential effects on the fetus.

Don't stop using contraception until you are ready to conceive! Some patients may believe that they are less fertile because of SLE, but that is not the case. Although certain medications, specifically high doses of steroids and the immunosuppressive drug cyclophosphamide (Cytoxan) may adversely affect fertility in some patients, most will not have any more difficulty conceiving than other women. (During times of a severe flare, women often experience menstrual irregularities, where their periods decrease in number or disappear completely. However, even during these times, you can't count on being infertile.)

Your support system. Pregnancy exacts a steep physical and emotional toll on all prospective mothers but especially on SLE women. There will be times when you feel exhausted, anxious, and completely overwhelmed. You need to have relatives or friends on your side who can provide support. Prior to pregnancy, it is crucial to line up your team. Talk to your spouse, significant other, family members, and close friends about providing the extra help you may need during this special time.

Coping with the rigors of motherhood. Every woman who is considering pregnancy needs to do a bit of soul searching. Although most women will fare well, some will become ill during or after pregnancy. In fact, in some cases, once the baby is born, the mother may be too sick to care for her child. If a woman has severe SLE, she may have frequent flares as the child is growing up, which may hamper her ability to be an effective parent. If a woman is frequently feeling exhausted and fatigued without children, she is going to feel even more overwhelmed by the hard work of raising children. Before a woman decides to have a child, in fairness to herself and her child, she should consider whether she will be able to take care of that child at least most of the time. If possible, she should plan to have some extra help right after the baby is born to give her some time to regain her strength. She also needs to begin thinking about setting up a network of family, friends, or hired help who will help her on days that she may not feel up to the rigors of parenting.

Financial considerations. If you're part of a two-paycheck family or if you're self-supporting, you need to consider the fact that pregnancy and motherhood could hamper your earning potential. If you experience a flare during pregnancy, you may be unable to work. In addition, after childbirth, you may have a rougher time juggling a job with parenthood, especially if fatigue is a problem.

Medical insurance. The cost of prenatal care and delivery can be very high, especially for a mother who may require extra care or an infant who needs to spend time in an intensive care nursery.

Check your medical insurance policy to make sure that you have adequate coverage.

WILL MY BABY BE HEALTHY?

Perhaps the most important question of all is, Will my baby be healthy? In most cases, the answer is unequivocally yes. Although there is some familial risk in developing a connective tissue disease, the vast majority of children born of SLE mothers will not have lupus. However, there are some problems that may crop up during pregnancy and beyond.

About half of all babies will be carried to term and will be completely healthy, robust infants. Studies have shown anywhere from 25 to 50 percent of all SLE pregnancies will result in miscarriage or stillbirth. The 33 percent of lupus women with antiphospholipid antibodies run a greater risk of developing complications during pregnancy that can adversely affect the fetus. These antibodies may cause blood clots in the placenta that prevent the placenta from developing normally and providing adequate nutrition to the growing baby. In many cases, with proper treatment, however, the problem can be controlled. In general, good prenatal care can greatly reduce the risk of fetal loss, although it is still going to be somewhat higher than normal.

Women with SLE run about double the risk of delivering premature babies—about 20 percent will deliver before 37 weeks. Although prematurity can result in many serious and potentially life-threatening health problems for the infant, prompt medical attention can prevent many of these problems. In addition, an educated mother can work with her obstetrician to prevent premature delivery.

About 30 percent of all women with SLE test positive for Ro antibody. Between 5 and 10 percent of these women will give birth to babies with neonatal lupus, usually characterized by a rash, photosensitivity to sun, sometimes fever, and a low platelet count. Neonatal lupus typically disappears within three to six months, when the maternal antibody is out of the baby's system. If a mother with Ro antibody has had a baby with neonatal lupus, she stands a 25 percent chance of having another with a subsequent pregnancy.

About half of all infants born with neonatal lupus will have congenital heart block, a permanent condition that will result in a slow heartbeat. Fortunately, these children can be treated quite successfully with a pacemaker, a mechanical device that can be implanted in the chest to speed up the heart rate to normal levels.

Recent studies show that a small percentage of children with neonatal lupus may develop some form of connective tissue disease later in life; however, most will not.

WHAT ABOUT FLARES?

One of the most controversial issues surrounding SLE is whether or not pregnancy can cause flares. Those who believe that SLE is caused by the body's inability to metabolize estrogen normally feel that pregnancy, a time of hormonal turmoil, must surely wreak havoc on SLE women. Frankly, the studies are quite contradictory. One well-done study followed women during pregnancy and for a year postpartum. The result: There was no evidence that women had more flares during pregnancy than during the year following pregnancy. In fact, a handful of women actually went into remission. However, another study performed at Johns Hopkins Medical School found that pregnancy did indeed trigger flares in many women. Why the different findings? The study with the good result was of women at a special SLE clinic at a major New York hospital. These women were, for the most part, getting excellent care prior to and during the pregnancy. On the other hand, the women at Johns Hopkins were mostly poor inner-city women who may not have had access to good medical care before getting pregnant. These studies underscore the importance of maintaining good health prior to conception.

One bright note: The majority of women who experienced flares during pregnancy did not get seriously ill. Most women had mild symptoms, including joint pain, skin rashes, and excess fatigue.

About 20 percent of all lupus flares during pregnancy are to women who were previously undiagnosed with SLE. These new cases tend to be more serious than flares in women who have a history of lupus.

Women who terminate their pregnancies through therapeutic

abortion may also be at increased risk for flares. Perhaps these women are sicker to begin with, which is why they opt for abortion, or the flares may be caused by hormonal changes.

If a woman does flare during pregnancy, she can be safely treated with appropriate doses of certain steroids (prednisone, prednisolone, and methylprednisone) that are broken down in the placenta before reaching the fetus. (If a woman takes steroids during pregnancy, immediately after delivery the physician should check the baby's glucose and electrolyte levels as well as adrenal gland function.) Low-dose aspirin is believed to be safe; however, it must be stopped 2 weeks prior to delivery. Hydroxychloroquine (Plaquenil) should probably not be given during pregnancy because it may cause eye damage to the fetus and may also suppress the fetal immune system. Of the immunosuppressive drugs, azathathioprine (Imuran) has been successfully used in many seriously ill women and is believed by many experts to be safe for pregnancy. (Check with your physician before taking any medication during pregnancy.)

PLANNING FOR PREGNANCY

Once you decide that you are physically and emotionally ready for motherhood, the next step is to line up the medical team that will see you through the pregnancy. In addition to your primary care physician, a woman with SLE should be treated by a high-risk obstetrician who has had experience in handling lupus pregnancies. Because of the problems that can arise for both mother and baby, the obstetrician should be affiliated with a well-respected, modern medical facility with a state-of-the-art neonatal intensive care nursery. Home birth, a birthing center, or a neighborhood hospital without a neonatal intensive care nursery is out of the question for most women with SLE.

I think it's a good idea for you to meet with your high-risk obstetrician before pregnancy to discuss your particular case. The obstetrician will review your overall medical history as well as any miscarriages, stillbirths, or past pregnancies that might portend the outcome of future pregnancies. Keep in mind that even if you've had previous fetal loss, it doesn't mean that your next pregnancy won't be successful, but it does mean that you may require special treatment. Although protocols may vary from doctor to doctor, most high-risk obstetricians will suggest that their new SLE patients undergo the following blood tests prior to conception. Many of these tests will be redone at various points during the pregnancy to track the health of the mother and baby.

✦ PLATELET COUNT. Platelets are clotting cells that help prevent bleeding. Around one-third of all SLE patients will develop a low platelet count during pregnancy. It's important to establish a baseline platelet count prior to conception. A decline in platelets could indicate a complication in the pregnancy, including preeclampsia, a potentially life-threatening disease for mother and baby, or lupus flare.

✦ URINANALYSIS AND 24-HOUR URINE COLLECTION. The urine is tested for protein and creatinine to assess the function of the kidneys. The physician will also look for signs of red or white blood cells in the urine, which could indicate inflammation. Kidney disease is usually symptomless; therefore, this test is the only way to determine the health of the kidneys. It is also important to establish a baseline for protein; during pregnancy, protein in the urine can be a sign of preeclampsia.

✦ COMPLEMENT LEVEL. Complement components are a series of proteins in the blood that are involved in the inflammatory process. A low complement level prior to pregnancy could indicate active disease. During pregnancy, a drop in complement could signal a flare or an increase in disease activity.

✦ ANTIPHOSPHOLIPID ANTIBODIES. Patients with a high titer of IgG anticardiolipin and/or the lupus anticoagulant are at risk of developing blood clots that result in small, undergrown placentas. As a result, the fetus may be denied adequate nourishment. These women are at greater risk of miscarriage, usually during the second trimester, and stillbirth. Throughout their pregnancies and postpartum period, some women with antiphospholipid antibodies are also at greater risk of developing deep-vein thrombosis, or clots in their legs or elsewhere in the body. Interestingly, many women with these antibodies have normal pregnancies.

✦ TEST FOR RO AND LA ANTIBODIES. Women with these antibodies are at greater risk of giving birth to children with neonatal lupus syndrome and congenital heart block.

✦ TEST FOR INFECTION. Women with SLE may be more prone

to developing certain infections that could harm the fetus. If you have a history of abnormal Pap smears or a history of genital herpes infection, your doctor may want to test you for any current infection.

During pregnancy, your physician may order additional tests to keep track of you and your baby's progress. Here is a partial list of some of those tests and what they may reveal.

✍ ULTRASOUND (SONOGRAM). Sound waves of extremely high frequency are bounced off the fetus to produce a picture or sonogram of the fetus on a screen or monitor. From this sonogram, the physician can evaluate the size of the placenta, assess the growth of the baby, and examine the fetal heart for potential abnormalities. Sonograms are usually performed every trimester but may be done more often if the physician suspects a problem.

✍ ALFA-FETOPROTEIN TEST. This blood test, which is usually performed at 16 weeks after conception, measures the amount of alfa-fetoprotein, a protein formed in the liver of the fetus and is also present in smaller amounts in the mother's blood and amniotic fluid. A higher than normal level could indicate a possible birth defect of the neural tube, such as anencephaly or spina bifida. Women with SLE frequently test abnormally high for alfa-fetoprotein, although they are at no greater risk of having babies with neural tube problems. In SLE women, however, a higher than normal result is associated with a greater risk of preterm delivery.

✍ FETAL MONITOR OR NONSTRESS TEST. The nonstress test is a noninvasive procedure that is performed after the 24th week to measure fetal activity. A belt or monitor is placed around the mother's abdomen as she rests on the examination table. (This test is usually performed in the doctor's office but may be done at a hospital.) The monitor is linked to a machine that records fetal activity on a printout, similar to an EKG. This test records fetal heartbeat after activity; after each burst of activity, the heart should speed up. If the heart rate is slow or sluggish, it could be a sign of a fetal problem, such as infection or malnutrition from an inadequately functioning placenta.

✍ BIOPHYSICAL PROFILE. Performed after the 24th week, the biophysical profile can assess the overall health of the fetus. This procedure includes a sonogram as well as a nonstress test. From this test, the physician can obtain important information, such as the amount of amniotic fluid, which will indicate whether the fetus is being adequately nourished; the frequency and type of fetal movement; and the position of the baby—a healthy baby will be in a tightly packed fetal position while an ailing baby will appear limp and flailing. If the biophysical profile reveals that the baby is in danger, the physician may opt for surgical or induced delivery.

MONITORING YOUR PREGNANCY

As a high-risk obstetrical patient, you will have to make more frequent visits to your physician and will be monitored more closely. However, most of the time, you will be on your own, and therefore it is of critical importance that you alert your doctor to any signs of trouble as early as possible. For women without SLE, it is often difficult to distinguish the usual aches and pains of pregnancy from the more serious signs of trouble. It is even a more challenging task for women with SLE who may be used to some degree of chronic discomfort. To help sort out the normal from the abnormal is the following list of some of the common bodily changes that occur during pregnancy as well as those that should be taken as potential threats.

WHAT TO EXPECT

Mild swelling. Most women will have some mild swelling, especially around their ankles.

Morning sickness. Occasional bouts of nausea and vomiting are normal during the first trimester.

Frequent urination. Early in the pregnancy, hormonal changes may keep you running to the bathroom. Later in the pregnancy, the fetus may press down on the bladder, which will cause more frequent urination.

Skin changes. Women may notice that their pigmentation gets darker on certain parts of their body, such as their nipples, and they may develop a dark line down their abdomen. Some women develop a flush on their face and hands similar to the lupus rash.

Fatigue. Especially during the first trimester and the later part of the last trimester, women may feel very tired. Usually, women feel more energetic during the second trimester.

Indigestion and/or constipation. As the pregnancy progresses, many women become constipated or suffer from heartburn.

Fetal movement. By the 20th week of pregnancy, most mothers begin to feel some fetal movement.

Braxton-Hicks contractions. At around the 20th week, most women begin to feel occasional contractions called Braxton-Hicks, which prepare the uterus for labor.

Other annoyances. Occasional leg cramps, varicose veins, and hemorrhoids may occur, especially later in pregnancy.

WHAT MAY NOT BE NORMAL

If you experience any of the following, notify your physician immediately.

Bleeding or excessive bruising. Vaginal bleeding, spotting, or blood in the urine is never normal; it could be a sign of a threatened miscarriage or kidney disease. Bleeding gums or easy bruising could be a sign of low platelets.

Sudden weight gain. Gaining weight at the rate of a pound or two a week is to be expected, a sudden weight gain of more than two to three pounds a week could be a sign of another problem, such as kidney disease or preeclampsia.

Edema. Women with SLE may experience some swelling even when they're not pregnant. However, sudden swelling in the legs, hands, or feet or sudden puffiness around the eyes could be a sign of preeclampsia.

Abdominal pain. Abdominal pain could be a sign of many problems, some related to the pregnancy, some not.

Rash of unknown origin. It's not uncommon for SLE women to develop rashes. However, a rash is a very nonspecific symptom that could be caused by anything from German measles to Lyme disease to SLE. Therefore, if you suddenly develop a rash, call your doctor.

Severe nausea or vomiting. It's normal to feel somewhat queasy during pregnancy, especially during the first trimester. It is unusual to feel sick all the time and could be a sign of kidney disease.

Chills and fever. Chills and fever could be signs of infection.

Chronic exhaustion. It's normal for SLE women to feel fatigued at times, and it certainly is common for pregnant women to feel exhausted. However, severe, debilitating exhaustion could also be a sign of anemia or another problem.

Abdominal cramps. Depending on the stage of pregnancy, menstrual-type cramps could be a sign of miscarriage or preterm labor.

Feeling faint, dizziness, severe headache, blurred vision. Any of these symptoms could be a sign of preeclampsia, high blood pressure, diabetes, or other serious problem.

Gush of fluid from vagina. This could signify a leak in the amniotic fluid or the premature rupture of membranes, which could lead to premature birth.

Problems with urination. Burning or pain during urination, cloudiness in the urine, or blood in the urine should be reported to your physician. Most likely, it is a sign of a kidney or bladder infection, which can be quite serious during pregnancy.

Pain. Don't assume that every ache and pain is due to the pregnancy or due to lupus. A severe backache or unusual pain anywhere else in your body should be reported to your doctor.

Sudden decrease in fetal activity. After you begin to feel fetal movement (around the 20th week), you will begin to notice a pattern in your baby's activity level. Some are active at night, some may sleep during the day, and some may come alive during lunch. Whatever it is, make note of your baby's active periods. If you experience any dramatic slowdown or change in activity, for instance, a normally active fetus is quiet for several hours and does not respond to usual stimuli such as lying down or sitting up, call your doctor. It could mean absolutely nothing (your baby may have changed schedules), or it could be a sign that your baby is not getting adequate nourishment.

Preterm contractions. Although an occasional Braxton-Hicks contraction is normal, frequent contractions prior to term are not normal and could be a sign of preterm labor. If you frequently feel a sensation of tightening and relaxing of your abdomen, you may be having preterm contractions. Notify your doctor; he or she will be able to evaluate your situation.

POSSIBLE COMPLICATIONS

Fortunately, what can go wrong during pregnancy most often doesn't. Most women will have fairly uneventful pregnancies and healthy babies. However, there are some particular complications that can arise in a lupus pregnancy. Early treatment is the key to safeguarding maternal and fetal health.

LOW PLATELETS

About one-third of all expectant mothers with lupus will develop thrombocytopenia. A severe drop in platelets can result in abnormal bleeding and must be treated before delivery. A CBC, which should be performed several times throughout the pregnancy, will reveal thrombocytopenia, if present. The condition is usually treated with steroids, low-dose aspirin, or IV gamma-globulin. If detected and treated early, thrombocytopenia should not harm the health of either the mother or the fetus.

PREECLAMPSIA

Pregnant women with SLE are at twice the risk (14 percent) of developing preeclampsia, characterized by high blood pressure, excessive swelling, and protein in the urine, indicating a kidney malfunction. If untreated, preeclampsia can lead to eclampsia or toxemia, a potentially life-threatening condition characterized by convulsions, coma, and failure of major organ systems. Once detected, preeclampsia is usually treated very aggressively with antihypertensive medication to get the blood pressure down to normal levels. Given the similarity of symptoms of preeclampsia to an SLE flare, it is often difficult to distinguish one from the other. Certain laboratory tests may help the physician reach the correct diagnosis, but even they are not conclusive. In general, unlike a flare, the complement level does not usually dip during preeclampsia; however, in rare cases it might. In addition, red blood cells are usually not passed in the urine during preeclampsia, as they might be during a flare. Nor is the sedimentation rate elevated (a sign of inflammation) during preeclampsia, as it typically is during a flare. However, given the fact that there are always exceptions to the rules, the physician will probably decide to treat the woman for both possibilities. Typically, a woman with preeclampsia or a flare will be hospitalized and put on steroids and antihypertensive medication. In some cases, depending on the stage of the pregnancy and the health of the fetus and mother, premature delivery may be required.

BLOOD CLOTS

Women are normally at greater risk of developing blood clots during pregnancy, and SLE women run an even higher risk. In particular, women with antiphospholipid antibodies may develop clots in the placenta, which can lead to serious problems for the fetus, including premature delivery. However, just because someone has these antibodies does not mean that she is going to run into trouble; in fact, she has a 50 percent chance of having a perfectly normal pregnancy. Despite the risk, most doctors opt not to treat this problem unless a clotting problem has been present or there has been a previous miscarriage. Prophylactic treatment may be risky to the mother and fetus and, studies show, makes very little difference in the outcome of the pregnancy. If a clotting problem or miscarriage does develop, a physician may prescribe an anticoagulant (blood thinner) such as aspirin or heparin to prevent future formation of blood clots (coumadin is generally not used during pregnancy). In rare cases, the mother may be treated with immunosuppressive drugs or IV gamma-globulin. These treatments have not been fully studied for this condition, so no optimal treatment has been defined. As serious as the clotting problems may be, studies show that if a woman is closely monitored and treated at the first sign of trouble, she has an excellent chance of having a successful pregnancy.

PREMATURE DELIVERY

In the United States, about 10 percent of all babies are born prematurely, and that rate is double for lupus mothers. Prematurity can be very serious; it is responsible for 80 percent of all newborn deaths, and even if the baby survives, he or she can have serious health problems. If a woman is closely monitored throughout her pregnancy and takes good care of herself, she is less likely to develop the kind of emergency that leads to a premature or sudden delivery. And even if she is unable to carry to term, her physician may be able to plan for the premature delivery. For example, if there is enough time, special steroids can be administered to the mother that will cross the placenta and help the baby's lungs mature more rapidly or treat an inflamed fetal heart. However, there are times when it is absolutely necessary to perform an emergency delivery, and thanks to the growing sophistication of neonatal intensive care nurseries, premature babies can do very well.

TAKING GOOD CARE OF YOURSELF

Pregnancy is a time when a woman needs to take extraspecial care of herself, and this is doubly true for a woman with SLE. Pregnancy places your already stressed body under even more stress, and you need the physical and emotional stamina to cope. Getting enough rest is essential. All women feel tired during pregnancy; you may feel even more tired. Don't push yourself; rest when you need to. If you work outside of the home, find a quiet place to unwind and put your feet up during your lunch hour. Take a catnap when you come home from work. Don't wait until you feel exhausted; try to give yourself frequent respites throughout the day.

Good nutrition is also essential for both you and your developing baby. During pregnancy, a woman needs to consume roughly 300 additional calories daily to provide the extra energy, vitamins, and nutrients for her and her baby. Excessive weight gain, which can cause high blood pressure among other problems, should be avoided. It is especially important for SLE women to avoid gaining excess weight. After pregnancy, it can be very difficult to take off the extra pounds. In fact, the average woman permanently retains an additional seven pounds after each pregnancy! Women who are prone to gain weight, such as women on steroids, need to be especially vigilant about weight control during pregnancy.

It is also important to eat a sensible, well-balanced diet with adequate nutrition. Your physician will probably prescribe a multivitamin. However, pills cannot replace food. Following is a list of some essential vitamins and minerals that are often lacking from the diets of pregnant women.

ഡ FOLIC ACID. Prior to conception, and throughout your pregnancy, you need to be sure that you are getting enough of this important B vitamin (800 micrograms daily during pregnancy; 400 micrograms daily when not pregnant). Taken prior to conception and throughout pregnancy, folic acid greatly reduces the risk of neural tube defects in the fetus. Fortunately, folic acid is provided in most prenatal vitamins. (However, this doesn't do you any good if you're not taking these vitamins at conception.) To maintain an optimum level of folic acid, eat eggs, dark green vegetables, whole grains, and orange juice.

✍ CALCIUM. Pregnant women require 1,200 milligrams of calcium daily; prenatal vitamins provide between 15 to 25 percent of this mineral. If an expectant mother fails to take in enough calcium during pregnancy, she runs a greater risk of developing osteoporosis later in life. It is especially important for women with lupus to get enough calcium—they are already at greater risk for osteoporosis because of steroid treatment. In addition, calcium may help normalize blood pressure, which could theoretically decrease the risk of developing preeclampsia. Dairy products, green leafy vegetables, tofu, and canned salmon with bones are excellent sources of calcium.

✍ IRON. During pregnancy, when maternal blood volume grows dramatically, a woman needs between 30 to 60 milligrams of iron to ensure that she will be able to produce enough red blood cells for herself and the fetus. Women with SLE, who are prone to developing anemia, should be extra careful about taking enough iron. You don't need to develop iron-deficiency anemia on top of the anemia common to SLE! Iron deficiency will also contribute to exhaustion. Iron is included in most prenatal vitamins. Good food sources include red meat, peanuts, sunflower seeds, dark green vegetables, and whole grains.

✍ COPPER AND ZINC. Copper and zinc are present in many healthy foods and prenatal vitamins. Some studies suggest that these minerals may help prevent premature rupture of membranes, a major cause of premature birth. Zinc also helps keep the immune system functioning normally. Good sources of zinc are wheat germ and nuts. Good sources of copper include nuts and whole grain cereals.

WHAT TO AVOID

Women with SLE are advised not to smoke at any time, but during pregnancy, it is even more critical to heed this advice. Smoking can cause low-birth-weight babies and premature delivery, two problems to which lupus patients are already prone. In addition, all pregnant women should avoid alcoholic beverages even in small amounts, which can cause fetal brain damage, and recreational drugs of all kinds.

Watch your intake of salt, which can raise blood pressure in many people. Since high doses of some vitamins and minerals can be toxic, *don't take extra vitamin or mineral supplements without consulting with your physician.*

POSTPARTUM

As your hormones shift back to normal, your body undergoes many changes that will have physical and emotional ramifications. It's normal for all new mothers to feel tired, and some may feel a bit depressed. Hair loss, which can happen in SLE anyway, may occur following delivery or after discontinuing breast feeding. Usually, the hair loss seems worse than it really is, because during pregnancy, the hair appears thicker. Rest assured that for most women, within a year or so, the hair returns to normal thickness.

Try to get as much help as you can during this postpartum period. If you can't afford to hire help, enlist the assistance of your spouse, family members, or friends. Don't feel guilty or that you are an inadequate mother because you can't do it all yourself. Even women without SLE can be overwhelmed by the demands made upon them by a new infant.

Some women will flare during postpartum, and these women in particular will need extra support.

Breast feeding is a wonderful experience for new mothers and babies that promotes bonding and boosts the infant's immune system. Breast feeding is fine for women with SLE with the following caveats:

✆ PREMATURE BABY. A premature baby may not have the ability to suck adequately. Therefore, alternative forms of feeding may be required.

✆ LOW MILK SUPPLY. If your baby is premature or you are on steroids, you may not be able to produce enough milk.

✆ DRUGS. Medication can pass to your infant through breast milk. If you are taking high doses of aspirin or steroids (over 30 milligrams daily), Plaquenil, or certain immunosuppressive drugs, you should not breast-feed. If you're on low-dose steroids, be sure to breast-feed early in the morning prior to taking your medication. Allow four hours after your medication for the next breast feeding. (You may have to use a supplemental bottle.)

✒️ FATIGUE. Breast feeding can increase maternal fatigue. If you are exhausted to begin with, you may want to put your baby on a bottle as soon as possible.

Talk to your doctor about whether breast feeding is right for you.

CHAPTER 9

Living with Lupus

COPING WITH THE INITIAL DIAGNOSIS

After I was diagnosed with lupus, my doctor put me on prednisone. Within two days, I felt terrific. My body didn't hurt anymore, the fatigue was gone—I was my old self again. I went back to work, life got back to normal, and I pretty much forgot all about it. But about six months later, I began to feel sick again and my doctor said that the medicine wasn't working anymore. He put me on other medicine, and I did begin to feel better, but I got very depressed anyway. It finally sunk in what the doctor meant by "chronic illness"—it meant that this wasn't ever going to go away.

—Cindy, age twenty-seven

Being diagnosed with lupus can be an overwhelming experience for a patient and her family. It's not easy to accept the fact that you or your loved one may have a chronic illness, particularly one that does not follow any predictable course. Lupus is synonymous with

unpredictability. Even if you have mild disease, as most lupus patients do, you will still be living with the threat of a flare. And although you will probably be able to live a reasonably normal life,
you may be limited in certain ways that you would not be if you
did not have lupus.

All of this can be very hard to swallow, particularly for the typical lupus patient—a young woman—who is just beginning her
life as an adult. During a period when the world is supposed to be
full of possibilities and open doors, the young woman diagnosed
with lupus may see her world narrowing as doors are slammed in
her face. For the first time in her young life, she may be forced to
confront issues of mortality; she may fear becoming ill and dependent and being unable to fulfill her hopes and dreams.

Faced with the unpredictability of lupus, the newly diagnosed
lupus patient is often in a state of emotional turmoil not dissimilar
to the kinds of emotional swings experienced by people who have
suffered a traumatic loss, such as a death of a loved one, or have
been diagnosed with a terminal illness. In her book, *Death and
Dying*, Elizabeth Kubler Ross noted that grieving is a process con-
sisting of five distinct phases: denial, anger, bargaining, depression, and acceptance. I believe that patients who are diagnosed
with a chronic disease may experience similar feelings with some
important differences.

Initially, most patients deny the diagnosis. This is understandable: It is very difficult to accept that you have a disease, one for
which there is no cure.

The second stage, anger, is a normal reaction, particularly in
young patients who feel that they have been unfairly singled out to
bear this burden. While their peers are living normal lives—dating, going to work, and making plans—newly diagnosed lupus patients may feel that their lives are being consumed with blood tests
and visits to the doctor. They routinely ask, "Why did this have to
happen to me? What did I ever do to deserve this?" This anger is
often displaced; it may be directed at family members, close
friends, or medical professionals who just happen to be in the line
of fire.

Bargaining, making sweeping promises such as, If I get well, I'll
devote my life to helping the less fortunate, and other similar
promises, is another form of denial that many patients experience.

We like to believe that there is some rhyme or reason to the workings of the world and that someone "up there" is actually watching and making value judgments, and we have some way of controlling those judgments. Although there may be a higher force in the universe, unfortunately, illness is a random event that can happen to the best of human beings.

Depression, a feeling of helplessness and hopelessness, is also not uncommon, especially when the reality of the disease sinks in. Patients experiencing depression may become temporarily immobilized, unable to move ahead and make important decisions about their treatment programs or their lives. Fortunately, this rock-bottom depression often gives way to the final and most constructive stage: acceptance. The grieving spouse or the terminally ill patient has to accept the reality of a certain fate: death. The lupus patient has to accept the reality of an uncertain fate: living with the unknown. Only when you accept the situation, can you begin to devise the survival strategies that you will need to live a full and productive life.

Although each patient has to experience these stages in her own way, there are positive, constructive steps that she can take to help her cope.

◢ COUNSELING. Although some people may bristle at the notion that they need help, being diagnosed with a chronic illness is one of the most stressful events that can happen in life. To better help cope with powerful emotions such as anger and depression, patients can get counseling from a professional who is familiar with chronic illness. Ask your physician to refer you to someone he or she respects, or contact the Lupus or Arthritis Foundation for referral to a mental health professional, a psychologist or social worker who works with lupus patients.

◢ PEER SUPPORT. When you are diagnosed with a chronic illness such as lupus, you may feel very isolated and that your family, who you may normally turn to during times of crisis, do not understand what you are experiencing. But you don't have to go through this alone. Throughout the United States, local chapters of the Lupus Foundation and the Arthritis Foundation run self-help groups where people with SLE share information, experiences, and tips on coping. Keep in mind, however, that there may be people at the support groups who are a lot sicker than you. Do not immediately assume that you will end up like them. No two patients are alike, and another person's case is irrelevant to yours.

If you don't live near a support group or are too ill to get to one, you can call your local chapter of the Lupus Foundation of America to see if they can put you in touch with another patient with whom you can speak. In New York, patients can call LupusLine, a telephone hot line peer-counseling service run jointly by the Hospital for Special Surgery in New York and the Lupus Foundation. Every call is answered by another lupus patient who can provide emotional support and information (see Resources). Although support groups can be very helpful, be careful not to make the support group your only social activity. Although there may be times that you will be very preoccupied with your illness—during a flare or after learning of your diagnosis—it is unhealthy to allow your life to revolve around your disease.

❧ DEALING WITH CONCERNED FAMILY MEMBERS. A diagnosis of lupus doesn't just affect you, it can profoundly affect the people who love you. Your spouse may be terrified at the prospect of losing you to illness or at the increased responsibility he may have to assume in the home (see Chapter 7).

Your parents in particular will be very worried and concerned about you. In many cases, parents may have been the ones who cared for you when you were ill. At the time, you appreciated the home-cooked meals, the frequent calls, and the other offers of assistance. When you're feeling better, however, you may begin to feel as if you are being smothered by this attention. You need to be compassionate, understand their concern, and try to remember how your parents were there for you when you needed them. In most cases, once your parents recognize that you are well, they will back off.

For some parents, however, what began as legitimate concern may take the form of overinvolvement, and that is not healthy for either of you. Because lupus often strikes young women on the brink of adulthood, excessive parental involvement in their lives can resurrect the same issues that they confronted as they struggled for independence during adolescence. Relationships between parents and newly diagnosed SLE daughters can often be rocky. For example, one patient was being driven crazy by a mother who was calling her at work several times a day for the latest information on her condition and would demand weekly updates on her blood tests. After a while, the daughter began slamming down the phone in exasperation. "I was furious at her for constantly reminding me about my illness. To make matters worse, I was also feeling terribly guilty because of the impact my illness was having on my mother," this patient confessed.

You can avoid hurt feelings by setting limits early on. You are the one who has to decide how involved you want your parents to be in your medical life, and you need to be very specific in stating your needs. It is not unreasonable for you to tell your parents, "I love you, but I don't want to talk about lupus all the time. I don't want to have to report to you and Aunt Agnes my ANA and creatinine levels each week. I don't want my lupus to be the main topic of discussion at every family dinner. I'll tell you when something important happens or when I need something."

If your parents are anxious to help, let them channel those feelings in a positive way. It can be helpful if parents ask directly what they can do to help. The parents who are the most constructive are the ones who say, "Look, we're here for you. Tell us if you need someone to drive you to the doctor or baby-sit or if there is anything else that we can do to help you." Parents with resources may be able to offer financial support, which may be necessary, particularly if their daughter is unable to work. Both the patient and her parents should keep in mind that she may be needier during times of illness and may need to assert her independence during the times when she feels well.

Family members should not interfere with the patient's relationship with her doctor unless they feel that the doctor is placing their loved one's health at serious risk. It does no good to try to second-guess the doctor or to alarm the patient by saying things like, "Aren't steroids very dangerous?" or "Did your doctor really say you could still keep working?" The patient–doctor relationship is an important one, particularly in the case of a chronic illness where they will be working together for a long time. If a patient has a question or is troubled by something the doctor is doing or saying, she should make the doctor aware of her concerns or get a second opinion. However, it is wrong for third parties to chip away at the patient's confidence in her physician unless it is for a very good reason.

Well-meaning parents may also become overprotective of their daughters to the point that they are actually causing harm. After the initial diagnosis, some parents may try to curtail their daughter's activities and may discourage them from doing anything that they believe is too strenuous. As one patient noted, "My parents and I really came to blows after I was diagnosed. If I mentioned that I wanted to do something or I was going somewhere, my mother would tell me not to do it. She believed that there had to be certain restrictions on my life, but I desperately wanted to try to live as normal a life as possible. When she saw that I was capable of doing a lot more than she thought, she finally stopped trying to run my life."

If parents are advising you against doing something that is clearly dangerous—skydiving, bungee jumping, hitchhiking cross-country—yes, you should listen to them and try to find out why you may be attracted to doing inappropriate things. However, if you want to pursue normal activities, like going back to school, working, or even taking a well-planned trip, it's a different story. If you feel capable of doing something, and your physician doesn't object, you have to follow your own best instincts. There are times that you may be limited by lupus, but it's a mistake to automatically assume that you can't live a normal life.

✎ WHO TO TELL. When you are first diagnosed with lupus, you should be fairly selective about who you tell. Many times, patients will come into my office very upset because of a thoughtless comment made by a friend or acquaintance about a friend of a friend who died a horrible death from lupus. If you mention any disease, lupus included, someone will have a scare story that they're just dying to tell. Although you may know deep down inside that gossip isn't fact, these stories may still be disturbing. In addition, well-meaning people may begin to get overly involved in your life. You should only discuss lupus with people who can contribute to your life in a positive way.

✎ MAINTAIN YOUR GOALS. You may be diagnosed with lupus, but lupus should not be your entire life. Staying home and focusing on your every ache and pain is bad medicine. It is not good for you or your family. You need to make plans, have goals, and get on with living life to its fullest. You may think, Well, that sounds like great advice, but how can I plan? I can flare at any time. I could end up a lot sicker. Although this may be true, keep in mind that even if you do flare periodically, flares pass. In all probability, you will not be in a state of acute illness all the time. It is of great importance that you try to achieve your goals; you are likely to be successful. But even if you fail, it may not be due to lupus. There are literally countless reasons why people do not fulfill their dreams, and illness is just one of them. As you learn to live with this disease, you will gradually learn your limits and what you can and cannot do. But don't make the mistake of setting arbitrary limits for yourself. As one lupus patient, an attorney in New York, so eloquently put it, "If you get a disease like lupus, and you get depressed, what are you depressed about? You're depressed because you think that your life is going to be wrecked, that nothing is going to be the same. If you waste one second not leading the best life that you can lead, then you're just as bad as the disease. You've destroyed your life just like the disease might have done."

❧ AVOID SELF-CENTEREDNESS. Although I stress throughout this book that you have to take good care of yourself, it is also important to be sensitive to the needs of others. When you have a chronic illness, there is always a risk of becoming overly self-involved and wrapped up in your own problems. This will only make things worse. It is essential to maintain some kind of perspective and worldview. Keep in touch with the outside world as much as possible. Read the newspaper, stay current with what's happening in your community. It's essential to be able to talk and think about something other than your illness. You also need to listen to other people—you're not the only one with problems. Be a good friend; keep track of what's going on in the lives of people that you care about. Don't forget to ask about their jobs, their children, and whatever else is important to them. Remember to acknowledge birthdays and other important life-affirming events. If you're totally self-involved and fail to reach out to others, they will quickly tune you out.

It's reasonable to expect help when you are sick and can't perform certain tasks. It is also reasonable to expect you to offer help to others when you are well. If a friend or neighbor has been particularly kind or considerate, think of ways to reciprocate. If your parents have gone out of their way to be available when you need them, try to be available to them when they need you. If women at the lupus support group provided strength when you were down, when you're feeling strong, go back to the group and be a shoulder for someone else to lean on. Get active in your church or synagogue. You will find that helping others can be very therapeutic.

MANAGING YOUR LIFE

I think that needing help, not being able to do it all yourself, is a big issue for American women. We're supposed to do a lot of different things and be good at all of them. Even Hillary Clinton is supposed to bake cookies while she's pushing through health care reform.

—Ellen, lupus patient,
mother of two, with a full-time job

If you're going to live as full and active a life as possible, you're going to have to develop your management skills. Specifically, you will have to learn how to manage your time well, how to manage other people well, and how to manage the emotional conflicts that typically arise in women when they can't be everything to everybody.

Women today are under a great deal of pressure. We are expected to work outside the home, raise a family, and run the household single-handedly. (Whether we work or not, in most cases, women are still responsible for child care and the bulk of the housework.) Healthy women without a chronic disease have been known to buckle under these strains. It is doubly difficult for a woman with lupus, who may have the same responsibilities but less energy. There are days when you may wake up feeling stiff and more tired than when you went to sleep. There are afternoons when you may be overcome by fatigue or suddenly hit with a fever. If you try to do too much at one time, you may have to pay by spending the next few days in bed. Therefore, it is very important that you learn to maximize your efficiency so that you can do what you need to do without getting yourself sick.

☙ GET ENOUGH REST. The first and primary rule is not to let yourself get exhausted. Get enough sleep at night. Although spending the day in bed isn't recommended unless you are very sick, naps can be a godsend. A 20-minute catnap in the afternoon or early evening can refresh you for the evening, particularly if you've spent the day caring for children or working in an office. If you have children at home, rest when they can watch their favorite television show or video. If you work outside of the home, get your family used to the idea that you are going to take your shoes off, close your bedroom door, and take a brief rest before preparing dinner. (They can begin making preparations without you.) Try not to let anything interfere with your naps—rest is good preventive medicine.

✿ SET PRIORITIES. Most women—with or without lupus—try to do too much in a given day. When tasks go unaccomplished, we feel frustrated and angry at ourselves. This is not only placing an unfair burden on us, but is counterproductive since frustration can sap us of our energy. Therefore, we all need to learn how to be realistic about our expectations. Setting daily priorities can be a big help. Every day, write a list of what you feel absolutely needs to be accomplished. After finishing your list, try to pare it down by at least 50 percent. Although this may sound difficult, once you begin thinking about what's truly necessary and what isn't, you will find that the list quickly shortens. For example, ask yourself, Do you really need to go grocery shopping in the evening, or can you wait another day or two? Can you call the store for a delivery? Do you have to bake cookies for your child's school or can you buy them instead? Do you have to do the laundry every day, or can it wait? Learning to set priorities can be an invaluable skill.

✿ LEARN YOUR LIMITS. It is equally important to learn that regardless of what may need to be done, there are times when you simply can't do it. As one patient put it, "There are times when I feel so tired that I know if I push myself, I'll only get worse. On those days, I ask myself, 'What is the most important thing that I have to do today?' Sometimes, it's sitting quietly and reading a book to my daughter—it's a little thing, but it means a lot to her. I don't worry about the dishes, the laundry, or anything. Usually, I'll feel better the next day and can finish what I need to do."

✿ ASK FOR HELP. Before you get exhausted, before you feel like an emotional wreck, ask for a helping hand. If you're living in a house with other people, you should be able to assign them tasks. Children can help clear the table, take out the garbage, or throw the laundry in the machine. Your husband can help around the house, particularly on days when you may be out of commission. If you're lucky enough to be able to hire household help, do so.

Be direct with other family members about asking for what you want. Very often, women make the mistake of believing that their husbands or children should somehow be able to read their minds and anticipate their needs. When their loved ones do not come through for them, they are terribly disappointed. It's far better for everyone to let people know what is expected of them.

ᏭᏮ LOOK FOR THE EASY WAY. If you've ever looked into the kitchen of a fast-food restaurant, you will see efficiency at work. All the supplies and cooking utensils are strategically placed so that the chefs and servers do not have to take one extra step or make one extra movement to slow them down. You need to adopt some of these practices in your life, not for speed, but for energy conservation. Think of how you can organize your surroundings to make life a bit less wearing. This will take some imagination, but once you get the swing of it, it's quite easy. For example, if your washing machine is in the basement down a steep flight of stairs, consider moving it somewhere else in the house. If that's not possible, you can try to minimize wear and tear by staying downstairs while the machine is going. Take the opportunity to enjoy some quiet time reading or listening to the radio. Or, if you have small children and find that you are constantly dragging their toys from the living room to their bedroom upstairs, leave a basket at the bottom of the stairs where you or they can deposit their toys after they're through playing. The Arthritis Foundation offers many different books and leaflets on energy conservation; call them to obtain these materials.

ᏭᏮ DON'T LEAVE THINGS FOR THE LAST MINUTE. The last thing you need to do is feel rushed and stressed. Therefore, it is critical that you learn to pace yourself so that you don't leave an important task or activity to the last minute. For example, I spoke with one mother who began organizing her two children's camp trunks in March, three months ahead of time. When June rolled around, both trunks were filled with the proper clothes, all labeled and neatly packed. This mother noted that she was able to perform this task at her leisure, without feeling pressured. However, if she had left it to the last week, as many of her friends with children had done, she would have been frantic. And when she gets frantic, she gets sick. Whatever the task—whether it's planning for a birthday party or preparing a report at work—try to start it as early as possible.

❧ BREAK DOWN BIG TASKS INTO LITTLE ONES. If you're faced with a job that seems overwhelming, try to figure out ways to break it down into smaller, more manageable tasks. For example, if you promised to bake your son a birthday cake but feel too tired at night to complete the job, do part of the job. Mix the dry ingredients in one bowl, the wet ingredients in another, and put them away in the refrigerator until morning. Then go to sleep and finish baking the cake the next day. Or if you feel the urge to clean your closet but can't summon up the energy to do it all at once, clean out a small portion of it, and do the rest later or on another day.

❧ CONTINGENCY PLANNING. If you are at the hub of a busy household and a lot of people rely on you, you need to plan for days when you simply can't do your job. Don't wait for the emergency to happen; have your plan in place. Make a list of friends, relatives, and neighbors who will agree in advance to drive the car pool, make the kids' lunches, or baby-sit for small children if you feel too sick to even get out of bed. Ideally, your list should include several names so that you aren't always imposing on the same person. However, in some cases, a sibling, parent, or in-law may be more than happy to be on call. If you don't have that kind of support system, however, you'll have to create one. If you can afford it, you may be able to hire help from a home care or baby-sitting service. If money is tight, check with local religious and civic organizations to see if they offer any free programs for emergency assistance. If you live near a chapter of the Lupus Foundation, perhaps you can organize a network of women who will help each other out when one of them is not feeling well. Although developing a contingency plan may take time and energy, it is well worth the effort.

TIPS ON COPING WITH CHILDREN

Since lupus typically strikes during the childbearing years, many women with lupus are also mothers. Raising a child is not easy under any circumstances—it is both physically and emotionally demanding—and it can be especially difficult if you have physical limitations due to illness. It may take every ounce of your energy to make it through the day, even if you have a supportive spouse who does his share of child care. For a single mother, it is even more difficult.

A mother's illness can also have a profound impact on her child. Nevertheless, there are many functioning mothers with lupus who are raising healthy and happy children. Although it is certainly possible for the children of lupus mothers to have fairly normal childhoods, it's important to understand that these children—whether they show it or not—are also under particular forms of stress. Clear and open communication between parent and child is the key to overcoming these potential problems.

WHAT TO TELL THE CHILDREN

If your disease is "in remission," and lupus doesn't affect your life in any way, there's no need to worry small children by telling them that someday in the future you may get sick. At some later date, you may explain to an older child that you have lupus and what it is, but as long as you seem perfectly healthy, there's no reason to bring up the subject.

However, if you have obvious symptoms, such as fatigue, fevers, or joint pain, your child will notice that you're not well. Some may ask directly, "Are you sick, Mommy?" Others may not say anything but may fear that you are sicker than you really are. It's far better to tell children the truth than to keep them guessing. Simply say, "Mommy has an illness that sometimes makes her feel bad. Although I may look very sick, it's not very serious. And there are plenty of days that I feel just fine." If there are particular parts of your body that hurt, let the child know. Children can be surprisingly understanding. As one mother explained, "My little one was three when I was diagnosed. From the beginning I told him that there are days when Mommy gets bad headaches or when you can't go jumping on Mommy's lap because my legs hurt. I just say, 'Eric, it's not a good day for you to jump all over me. But you can give me a hug and I'll be very happy.' And most of the time, I don't have to tell him more than once."

No matter how you may minimize your lupus, your children may fear that you are going to die. Children between the ages of four to eight are especially concerned about death and may ask you periodically, "Is Mommy going to die?" Reassure them that although you may seem sick at times, people with lupus can live a very long lifetime.

The worst thing that you can do is to try to hide your lupus. If a child sees you grimacing in pain and taking medicine, she will know that something is wrong. If you deny what she sees, she will find it very confusing. She may even believe that somehow she is responsible for making you feel bad.

As children mature, they may wonder whether they will get lupus also. Make sure that they understand that the odds are they will not. Although there is a very slight chance that they may develop lupus or some other autoimmune disease, I would certainly not alarm them.

UNDERSTAND THEIR ANGER

Having a mother who is chronically ill is not the norm. Your children will see other mothers doing many things that you can't do, and they may become angry at you for your "deficiencies." They may resent the fact that you are "always napping" or they can't invite other children over at a moment's notice because you may be having a bad day and you just don't have the strength to supervise other children. Although you can expect children to be somewhat considerate of your needs, there are limits to their understanding. They are just children and can't be expected to behave with adult maturity. Don't make them feel bad or guilty for being angry, instead acknowledge how they feel. Say directly, "I know that you're angry because when I'm sick, Tommy can't come over to play. I'm sorry that I don't feel well, but I can't help it. When I'm well, I promise I'll take you and Tommy to the movies." When you feel better, be sure to deliver on your promise!

In some cases, angry children may act out in school or with other children. If your child's grades begin slipping or you begin to get reports that your previously well-behaved youngster is getting into fights or other trouble at school, it may be a sign that he is having difficulty coping. In these situations, parents may consider professional counseling for the child and the family. The school guidance counselor, the Lupus Foundation, or the social work department at your local hospital may be able to refer you to the appropriate individual or organization.

DEALING WITH ENERGETIC CHILDREN

When you're feeling exhausted or your body hurts, caring for an energetic toddler or child who is bouncing off the walls can be very trying. During these times, consider taking your child to a play group—either at another mother's home or run by a community center or local Y—or a supervised program such as Gymboree. In a play group, the child will be distracted by other children and will not require your total attention. At a preschool or supervised program, your child can burn up some energy in a fairly safe environment.

SPEND TIME TOGETHER—NO MATTER WHAT

Even when you're sick, it's of critical importance to spend time with your children. Figure out a time when you feel the strongest—maybe it's late morning or after a nap. If you can muster up the strength, you can play a game, take a walk, or do a special activity. If you're too tired to play with your children, you can read to them (or if they're older, they can read to you), play cards, or even cuddle in bed and watch a video together. The most important thing is that your children feel that you love them and that they are not shut out from your life.

STAY INVOLVED IN THEIR LIVES

Being an involved concerned mother is not only good for your children, it's good for you. You don't want to become so involved in your illness that you begin to shut out the people who love you. If you are sick, you may not be able to be Little League coach or troop leader for the Girl Scouts, but there are other things that you can do. (By the way, if you're well or have mild disease, there's no reason why you can't do either of these things.) When you're feeling up to it, volunteer to work at the school library for an hour or two a week, help at the annual school bake sale, or help organize the class Christmas party (most of the work can be done over the phone by enlisting the aid of other mothers). Try to choose "high-profile" activities that show your children that you can be like any other mother.

DON'T OVERBURDEN YOUR CHILDREN

As your children get older and are capable of doing more things around the house, it is perfectly reasonable to expect them to help out. Children can be in charge of such chores as doing laundry, keeping their rooms neat, and baby-sitting on occasion for younger siblings. There are times when you are sick that a child may be called upon to take more responsibility. However, it is unfair to routinely overburden children with chores to the point that they can't participate in extracurricular activities or don't have time to do their main job—their schoolwork. A child should not be expected to cook dinner every night, do the shopping, or be used as a primary source of child care for younger siblings. A child should not be the surrogate mother: If your household is becoming overly dependent on a child to keep it afloat, you need to look for other sources of help. Could your spouse do more around the house? Is there a parent or another relative who can pitch in? Can you pay someone to come in a few days a week to perform household chores? Try to imagine how you would manage if that child wasn't around.

COPING IN THE WORKPLACE

Today, many women not only have responsibility for running a household, but are breadwinners as well. There are a record number of women in the workforce, consequently, there are probably more women with lupus who are holding down jobs than ever before. They are in nearly every occupation, from law enforcement to health care to college administration. Like other women, many women with lupus are also working for both financial and emotional fulfillment. As one woman put it, "I love my job. I love getting out and being with other people. I know that if I wasn't working, I would focus on myself and my disease in a very negative way."

Most women with lupus, particularly those with mild disease, cope very well in the workplace and in most cases, they are able to perform their jobs well with few, if any, problems. In most cases, employers and co-workers are understanding and supportive if problems do arise. There are inspiring stories of co-workers banding together to help a colleague with lupus by doing such thoughtful things as doing her typing on days when arthritic symptoms made it too painful for her to move her fingers or bringing lunch to her desk on days when she was too tired to go out. I have heard stories of compassionate employers who have held jobs open for women who were hospitalized for months at a time. I have also heard tales of women in the midst of lupus flares who although they were homebound, set up computers and fax machines near their bedsides so that they would not fall behind in their work. In most cases, their efforts were greatly admired and appreciated by their employers and colleagues.

However, not all the stories have happy endings. There are women who have been fired when their employers found out that they had lupus or were not hired in the first place because the employers feared that they would get sick and run up excessive medical costs on the company health plan. Fortunately, this type of discrimination is no longer legal, thanks to the Americans with Disabilities Act of 1990, which became law in July 1992. Employers who do not comply with this law may be liable to pay compensatory and punitive damages as specified under Title VII of the Civil Rights Act of 1991. The ADA applies to most private employers and state and local governments; employers with fifteen or less employees are exempt and so is the federal government. The law specifically prohibits employers from discriminating against a qualified job applicant or employee solely on the basis of disability as long as the employee is able to perform the job with or without a "reasonable accommodation." Reasonable accommodation is defined as one that does not impose significant difficulty or expense. For example, an employer cannot refuse to hire a qualified person in a wheelchair simply because that person may require a different desk height than the other workers—raising or lowering a counter is certainly not going to be too difficult or expensive. However, an employer would probably not be required to undergo a major renovation simply to accommodate one person.

The law does not mandate an employer to hire a disabled person who does not meet the job qualifications or cannot perform the essential functions of the job. For example, if the job description calls for a degree in certified public accounting, the employer need not waive that requirement for disabled job applicants. Nor is the employer required to hire someone whose disability makes it impossible for her to do the job. For example, if lifting heavy objects is an essential part of a job, as in the case of a moving company, the employer would not be required to hire someone who is physically unable to perform this task. There are other aspects of the ADA that are important for anyone with a chronic illness. The following list reviews some important aspects of this recent change in the law and how it may affect you in the workplace.

∽ THE JOB INTERVIEW. An employer cannot ask a job applicant whether or not she is disabled or the severity of the disability. However, the employer can ask the applicant if she is able to perform the tasks of a specific job with or without reasonable accommodation. An employer can make a job offer contingent on the prospective employee submitting to a physical examination as long as all prospective employees are required to do so. The employer cannot reject an applicant based on the results of this medical examination unless the applicant's physical condition directly impairs her ability to perform the job.

∽ HEALTH INSURANCE. The ADA mandates that disabled workers have equal access to health insurance. However, it does not require employers to provide additional insurance for employees with disabilities. The employer cannot refuse to hire or fire someone because that person's disability (or the disability of a family member) may pose a financial burden on the company health plan. However, if the company insurance plan does not cover a particular disability or exempts preexisting conditions, the employer is not required to change its insurance carrier.

∽ ENFORCEMENT. If you feel that you've been discriminated against due to your disability, you must file a complaint with your local office of the U.S. Equal Opportunity Commission within 180 days from when the discrimination took place. Because the law is complicated, it's important to check with an attorney who specializes in employment law about your specific situation before filing your complaint. In addition, there are advocacy groups for the disabled that can provide information on your rights in the workplace (see Resources).

Another federal law, the Family and Medical Leave Act, which took effect in August 1993, may prove to be of benefit to women with lupus and their families. The law requires all employers with fifty or more workers to provide up to twelve weeks of unpaid leave during any twelve-month period to an employee who is ill or who must care for a sick spouse, child, or parent. The birth or adoption of a child is also covered under the law. The employee must be given her old job or an equivalent position upon returning to work. During the leave, the employee may not collect unemployment insurance or other government compensation. The employer must provide health care benefits during the leave. However, if the employee does not return to work, she may be liable to repay any health care premiums paid by the company during her leave.

The twelve-week leave can be taken in increments. For example, if you require special treatment such as kidney dialysis on a weekly basis, you may be able to arrange to take one day a week off as part of your nonpaid leave. In addition, if you are very ill, your spouse or parent may be able to take time off from their jobs to care for you or your children.

The downside of the Family and Medical Leave Act is that the leave is unpaid, therefore, many women who rely on their paychecks to make ends meet may be unable to take advantage of it. If you are ill and can no longer work, in some cases, you may be eligible for disability pay under Social Security. For more information, check with your local Social Security office or hospital social worker (see Resources).

Resources

CHAPTER 1

For general information on lupus, contact

Lupus Foundation of America, Inc.
4 Research Place, Suite 180
Rockville, MD 20850-3226
(800) 558-0121 (for written information)
(301) 670-9292 (for other questions)

Check your telephone directory for your local chapter. If it's not listed, call (301) 670-9292 for a list of regional chapters.

Arthritis Foundation
1314 Spring Street NW
Atlanta, GA 30309
(800) 283-7800

Check your telephone directory for your local chapter, or call or write to the national office in Atlanta for more information.

The American Lupus Society
3914 Del Amo Boulevard, Suite 922
Torrance, CA 90503
(310) 542-8891

Check your telephone directory for your local chapter, or contact the national office in California.

National Arthritis and Musculoskeletal and Skin Diseases Information Clearinghouse (AMS Clearinghouse)

Box AMS
9000 Rockville Pike
Bethesda 20892
(301) 495-4484

For emotional support and information, call Lupusline, which is
run by and for lupus patients under the auspices of the Depart-
mentment of Social Work of the Hospital for Special Surgery,
New York.

Lupusline
(212) 606-1952

CHAPTER 2

To locate a qualified rheumatologist in your area, call or write

American College of Rheumatology
60 Executive Park South, Suite 150
Atlanta, GA 30329
(404) 633-3777

For information on fibromyalgia, contact

Fibromyalgia Network
5700 Stockdale Highway, #100
Bakersfield, CA 93309

CHAPTER 3

For information on kidney disease, contact

The National Kidney Foundation
30 East 33rd Street
New York, NY 10016
(800) 228-4483

For information on cardiovascular disease, contact

The American Heart Association
7272 Greenville Avenue
Dallas, TX 75231-4596
(214) 373-6300

For information on Sjogren's syndrome, contact

Sjogren's Syndrome Foundation
382 Main Street
Port Washington, NY 11050
(516) 767-2866

CHAPTER 4

For information on medic alert identification, call or write

Medic Alert Foundation
PO Box 1009
Turlock, CA 95380
(209) 634-4917

For information on research and experimental therapies, contact

National Institute of Arthritis and Musculoskeletal and Skin Diseases of the National Institutes of Health
PO Box 9782
Arlington, VA 22209
(301) 496-8188

CHAPTER 5

For information on SPF clothing, call

Sun Precautions (FDA approved)
(800) 882-7860
Frogskin
(800) 354-0203
Solar Protective Factory
(800) 786-2562

CHAPTER 6

For assistance in quitting smoking, contact

Smokenders
(800) 828-4357

To find a specialist in treating addictions, contact

The American Society of Addiction Medicine
12 West 21st Street
New York, NY 10010
(212) 206-6770

For information on nutrition, contact

> **The American Dietetic Association**
> 216 West Jackson, Suite 800
> Chicago, IL 60606
> (312) 899-0040

For information on hair loss, contact

> **National Alopecia Areata Foundation**
> PO Box 150760
> San Rafael, CA 94915-0760

For information on cosmetics, contact

> **Covermark Cosmetics**
> 1 Anderson Avenue
> Monachie, NJ 07074
> (800) 524-1120

For up-to-date information on health advice and guidelines about immunization requirements for international travel, call

> **Centers for Disease Control and Prevention Hot Line**
> (404) 332-4559
> (fax)
> (404) 332-4565

For information on travel opportunities for the disabled, contact

> **Access: The Foundation for Accessibility by the Disabled**
> PO Box 356
> Malverne, NY 11565
> (516) 887-5798

CHAPTER 7

For information about sex and arthritis, read *Guide to Independent Living for People with Arthritis*. Atlanta: Arthritis Foundation, 1988.

This book is available from the Arthritis Foundation.

CHAPTER 8

For general information on pregnancy, contact

American College of Obstetricians and Gynecologists
409 12th Street SW
Washington, DC 20024-2188
(202) 638-5577

CHAPTER 9

For information on employment discrimination, contact

Eastern Paralyzed Veterans Association
75-20 Astoria Boulevard
Jackson Heights, NY 11370-1177
(718) 803-EVPA

Equal Employment Opportunity Commission
1801 L. Street NW
Washington, DC 29507
(202) 663-4900

For information on Social Security Disability Benefits, call the toll-free number (800) 772-1213 or get the following booklets from your local Social Security office:

⊷ *Disability* (SSA Publication No. 05-10029)

⊷ *When You Get Social Security Disability Benefits: What You Need to Know* (Publication No. 05-10153)

⊷ *SSI Supplemental Security Income* (SSA Publication No. 05-11000)

BIBLIOGRAPHY

Arthritis and Rheumatism: Abstracts of Scientific Presentations. Vol. 35, No. 9 (suppl.) (September 1992).

Arthritis and Rheumatism: Abstracts of Scientific Presentations. Vol. 36, No. 9 (suppl.) (September 1993).

Buyon, Jill P. Systemic lupus erythematosus and pregnancy. *Clinguide to Rheumatology*, Vol. 1, No. 4 (1991).

Carr, Ronald I. *Lupus Erythematosus: A Handbook for Physicians, Patients and Their Families.* Rockville, MD: Lupus Foundation of America, 1986.

Kelly, W., Harris, E., Ruddy, S., and Sledge, C. Eds. *Textbook of Rheumatology.* Philadephia: W.B. Saunders, 1993.

Klippel, John H. Ed. Systemic Lupus erythematosus. *Rheumatic Disease Clinics of North America*, Vol. 14, No. 2 (April 1988).

Lahita, Robert G. Ed. *Systemic Lupus Erythematosus.* New York: Churchill Livingstone, 1992.

Legato, M., and Colman, C. *The Female Heart: The Truth About Women and Coronary Artery Disease.* New York: Simon & Schuster, 1992.

Lewis, Kathleen. *Successful Living with Chronic Illness.* Garden City Park, NY: Avery Publishing Group, 1985.

McCarty, D., Koopman, W., Moore, M., McGrory, C., and Rosenthal, R. Eds. *Learning About Lupus: A User Friendly Guide*. Philadelphia: Lupus Foundation of Delaware Valley, 1991.

Phillips, Robert H. *Coping with Lupus*. New York: Avery Publishing Group, 1991.

Pitzele, Sefra Kobrin. *We Are Not Alone: Learning to Live with Chronic Disease*. New York: Workman Publishing, 1985.

Schumacher, H. Ralph, Ed. *Primer on the Rheumatic Diseases*. Atlanta: Arthritis Foundation, 1993.

Sergent, J., and Panush, R. Eds. Current controversies in clinical rheumatology. *Rheumatic Disease Clinics of North America*, Vol. 19, No. 1 (February 1993).

Talal, Norman. Ed. Systemic lupus erythematosus and Sjogren's Syndrome. *Current Opinion in Rheumatology*, Vol. 4 (1992).

Zurier, Robert. Ed. Pregnancy in patients with rheumatic diseases. *Rheumatic Disease Clinics of North America*, Vol. 15, No.2 (May 1989).

INDEX

Index